Mitton's *Practical Modern Herbal*

Mitton's
Practical
Modern
Herbal

F. and V. Mitton

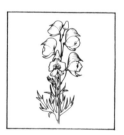 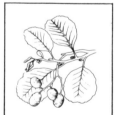 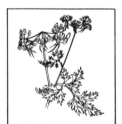

London

W. Foulsham & Co Ltd

NEW YORK TORONTO CAPE TOWN SYDNEY

W. Foulsham & Co. Ltd.,
Yeovil Road, Slough, Berks., England.

ISBN 0-572-00901-1
© F. and V. Mitton 1976
Art work © W. Foulsham & Co. Ltd. 1976

Printed in Hong Kong

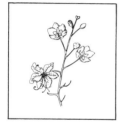

Contents

Foreword

The medicinal properties and effects of herbs are all well known because for countless thousands of years herbs were the only medication known to mankind.

Even today, when unparalleled advances have been achieved in medical science, many people still turn to herbal remedies, many of them ones which have been used and approved by their own parents, grandparents or even great grandparents.

This book has been written by people who have made the study of herbal medications their life's work. Although all quantities, methods and advice contained in this manual have been carefully checked, the authors and publishers do not hold themselves responsible for the resultant medicinal values. Should you be in any doubt about the safety of any of the medicines or herbs under consideration then the authors and publishers strongly recommend that you consult a qualified herbalist who will be in a position to study your individual symptoms and prescribe accordingly.

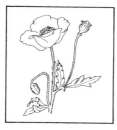

Preface

It is astonishing how few people know what a herbalist is. Most believe that he is a practitioner of primitive, superseded medical methods, in some way connected with witchcraft and magic; and many believe that he is an unqualified medical practitioner locked in illegal competition with the medical profession.

This is quite untrue. A herbalist's function is to procure and supply herbs to the public and nothing more. However, in actual practice it is necessary for him to advise potential users on the choice of herbs and methods of preparation, and, because these methods of preparation are often complex and difficult, to make available herbal products ready for a customer's use. Arising from this, standard formulation medicinal products are made in bulk to meet a constant demand. Thus, one may expect to enter any herbalist's premises and see displayed for sale a wide variety of products packed and ready for use.

Although one may suppose after reading the above paragraphs that a herbalist is a merchant, somewhat similar to a grocer, this is not so. A herbalist must be highly trained and competent, and above all vitally interested in the customer's problems and needs. His reputation, after all, is always built upon satisfied customers' recommendations. For this reason it is absolutely essential that he should know exactly what effects the herbs 'ie prescribes will have, and this is not just a matter of his personal genius or understanding.

The medicinal properties and effects of herbs are all exactly known, because for countless thousands of years herbs were the only medication known to mankind. Every primitive society and civilisation has contributed to the advance of herbal and medical science. Every continent and country has been combed and searched for plants with therapeutic qualities.

Mankind's most unremitting, unchanging desire has always been not power or wealth, but health and life itself.

The herbalist's basic training is the learning of the lore of the past, the understanding of the curative properties of plants and, of course, the identification and evaluation of herbal samples — he must **know**!

With this training it is obvious that the apprentice herbalist will experiment; but all experiments will be bounded by the precepts that a patient's health, or recovery, will not be jeopardized and that recovery will not be delayed. These experiments will all be developments of known herbal practice. Plainly expressed, the science of herbalism is a continuous process based upon the sure foundations of previous successful treatments. Indeed, it could not be otherwise. From the earliest Stone Age tribal medicine man to the present-day practitioners, herbalism has been a science — the first science in man's history. The world's first university, opened by the priests of Amun in the city of On in the Egyptian delta in 2000 BC, was concerned solely with the science of healing. The students were recruited from all parts of Egypt and resided in barracks built of dried mud and thatched with palm fronds, in the precincts of the great temple. The course lasted for four years and they defrayed the cost by working for five hours each day in the temple workshops, a practice that could well be re-introduced into our universities today! The training was standardized and students were taught to diagnose by question and observation, in much the same manner as they are today.

It is popularly supposed that these early doctors practised a mumbo-jumbo of worthless magic, but teaching manuals that have been discovered, written in hieroglyphs on papyrus rolls, prove that they were adept and skilful. They were also proficient dentists and were actually able to transplant living teeth!

Essential herbs were grown in well-tended gardens and dried in the Sun and in clay ovens; others not indigenous to the Nile settlements were imported with great difficulty and expense. The storage magazines for these valuable stocks were built of stone below ground to ensure an equable temperature, and were ventilated by air shafts. Many of the great pottery storage jars, each with the specific name of the contents painted on in hieroglyphs on the bulging shoulder, were found intact. One actually contained the dessicated remains of senna (**Cassia augustifolia**), used as a laxative and cathartic.

The remains of a processing shed were excavated nearby, and although the edifice had perished, the foundations and workbenches remained to surprise the archaeologists. The benches were constructed of polished limestone supported on brick piers. A ledge front and rear prevented the herbs from being brushed on to the floor and at intervals great mortars, worked from blocks of granite with polished working interiors, were set into the floor. It would seem that at least fifteen people could work at the benches, and the probable daily production of fresh ground herbs would have been about half-a-ton — a considerable turnover indeed!

These, the earliest mass-production medicinal manufacturers known, were just as efficient as manufacturers today. All of their products were packed in baked clay jars of uniform size and capacity. Each jar was impressed with a seal stating the contents and the date when consignments were carried up or down the Nile to the temples where they would be used.

Temple-trained practitioners were confident and competent. Amputations were skilfully carried out with the patient in a narcotics-induced stupor. Operations for the removal of cataracts were quite common, and successful treatments for the usual gamut of ills were abundantly reported in temple archives.

Although the medical practice of the ancient Egyptians is so well recorded, it is certain that they gained much of their knowledge from an even older civilization. The Sumerians, who settled in the alluvial lands between the Tigris and the Euphrates at some time around 4000 BC, perfected artificial irrigation and were the first people known to us to have developed writing and the ability to record abstract thought. (The system they devised is known as cuneiform.) They were also great traders, and their ships sailed right down the Persian Gulf and across to India, where they traded with the people of the Indus. Undoubtedly, the greater part of their cargoes, which had to be of high value to make the venture worth while, consisted of herbs. Established before the very dawn of history as the most wanted and valuable of exportable merchandise, medicinal herbs helped to create trade as we know it, and to spread civilization across the world.

Even today, the trading methods of the ancient Sumerian ship masters and merchants are almost unchanged. They were effective then and they are effective now. All that is different is the need. In Sumerian times, the world's total population was only about 40 million. Now it nears 2,000 million, fifty times as many. The areas in which herbal products can be gathered has decreased correspondingly. Wild ginseng roots (**Panax quinquefolium**) can no longer be collected in the accessible foothills of the Mongolian hinterland. This is now a rare and very, very valuable herb and a pound of the best root is worth $50.

But the demand increases. Although Man can land and drive about on the moon, or obliterate a great city and its people with one bomb, he cannot cure arthritis or even the common cold. Man's basic need remains — fifty-fold. Safe, effective, harmless herbal medication is still one of the most desired and necessary of all imported commodities, and will continue to be so in the foreseeable future.

Man needs herbal medication to assuage his ills, and the herbalist will never willingly fail him.

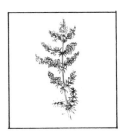

Part One

Herbal Medication
(Ancient and Modern Treatments — with reflections over twenty-one years of practice)

1. Why does it work?

The reason is simple. Because it is compatible.

Any material taken orally must pass into the stomach, where it will be broken down, assimilated into the bloodstream and circulated through the system, each organ retaining what is requires for its necessary functions. The process is relatively simple to understand from, let us say, an engineering viewpoint, but far more complex physiologically.

Since all animal and vegetable life is derived from a common form of life which originated in Archaeozoic times, about 4,000 million years ago, the molecular structure of each individual cell is similar, for the cells are the building blocks of life itself.

It is well to consider what a molecule is. Again the answer would seem to be simple, for we are informed that a molecule is a fixed pattern of atoms. The atom, modern science tells us, is a nucleus surrounded by rapidly orbiting electrons, rather like the familiar model of our solar system. Energy changes are manifested when an electron changes to a greater or smaller orbit. But now, the difficulty. It has recently been proved that the electron changes its orbit in no time at all, an impossibility in the material universe, and although it has the characteristics of a discrete source, it fills the entire sphere of its orbital diameter at once.

Thus, it becomes readily apparent that the simple particle picture of the atom is incorrect and that it must be regarded as something beyond the comprehension of our five senses. If this is so, then Man is unable to comprehend the microcosmos or, since all protoplasmic life forms are composed of atoms aggregated into molecular groupings, to understand life itself.

Without life, all matter is inanimate and insensible. Atoms combined into similar molecular structures but given life—even the lowest single-celled structures—are activated by a supreme motivation outside this space/time continuum that can only be the wish of a power greater than Man.

Complex life forms can sustain themselves only by consuming life forms. It is not possible for scientists to produce food from inanimate matter. Our bodies are sustained, thrive and reproduce by the assimilation of the food we eat, and this food is derived solely from the animal and vegetable kingdoms. We cannot exist upon inanimate matter, for it is incompatible and cannot be digested. Only vegetable life forms can, by utilizing the sun's energy to activate the process of photosynthesis, transmute inanimate matter into sugar and starches and sustain life.

Thus was established the life pattern of our planet more than 3,000 million years ago. The vegetable kingdom lives on the mineral resources and the animal kingdom lives on the vegetables. The two kingdoms, therefore, by virtue of common origin and kin, are compatible.

The ability of scientists now to synthesize drugs and food supplements from minerals is accepted as necessary, for there are insufficient supplies of herbal drugs to satisfy what has become an insatiable demand — and one that is taken for granted. Yes, taken for granted: an authoritative statement made by a scientist or a doctor is accepted simply because the vast majority of the public lack specialized knowledge to question it.

Now, why should herbal medication be effective? Simply, we believe, because we share a basic affinity with the vegetable kingdom. All vegetable matter, so long as it be not toxic or otherwise unfit for consumption, can be digested and excreted without any difficulty. Mineral matter, even if the molecular pattern is precisely similar, often cannot. The scientist's statement that a molecular pattern is 'precisely similar' is suspect, for rather should they say: "With the appartus and knowledge presently available, we believe the molecular patterns to be exactly similar, but there may be other circumstances of which we are not aware that can significantly alter this conclusion.'

A cloud of atoms combined into a molecule cannot be analysed or evaluated by any known process or understanding. Molecules in combination exhibit no discernible difference when examined in living or non-living forms, even if the patterns are considered similar. Indeed the virus, the smallest discovered self-reproducing unit, has yet to be proved to be a living organism.

So living organisms have an affinity with, and can profitably assimilate, other life forms, living or dead. There is a pattern that makes this possible, and that pattern is life. Herbal medication is indeed the medicine of life, and, provided it is taken after expert consultation and advice, it should give rise to no 'after' or 'side' effects.

In contrast, drugs synthesized from minerals or chemicals are known often to give rise to dangerous after, or, side-effects. There are several hundred children in Britain today who can attest to that. Unless long-continued, patient, expensive, expert research is carried out on the effects of drugs, the possible long-term effects cannot be known or mortality rates evaluated. Naturally, the scientists and manufacturers have to consider the time and capital to carry out this work—so there is danger in even the most respected man-made drugs, but it is extremely doubtful if these dangers will ever be found out!

Herbal medication is effective because countless generations of men have experimented with herbs and testified when the results have proved beneficial and warned when they have not. No other science can equal the proven evidence upon which scientific herbalism is based.

2. What is a man?

Man is a unique animal, because he uses miraculous intelligence to achieve worthless and dangerous results.

Man and the apes evolved from a common ancestor in Miocene times, but while the apes became highly specialized for life in the trees, Man ventured into the grasslands and open spaces and had to learn a new way of life. The earliest men whose fossil remains we can study are known as **Australophithicus.** They were omnivorous feeders who remained in family groups for reasons of safety. These first men were quick and agile, and were blessed with quick-focusing, perceptive vision and acute hearing, but they lacked the strength to become predators. Thus they became foragers, forever handling and searching, so that as the generations passed they evolved into men with powers of reasoning and learned to use stones and sticks as tools.

This was the step forward in evolution that marked the parting of the ways between Man and animal. From then on these primitive ancestors of ours, armed with stones chipped into hard axes, clubs and untipped spears, were, when they hunted in coherent bands, the masters of the world.

It was at this point that the personal sense of identity and ownership began to take form. Men became the first animals in evolutionary history to become aware of themselves as individuals, the first to claim ownership, and the first to defend their property for motives they could intelligently understand. As speech was developed it became possible to pass this knowledge on to children within a tribe.

Thus, over a million years ago in the Pleistocene age, Man had developed into an aggressive, acquisitive, thinking animal, and these personal characteristics have given him dominion over the earth. While he possesses them, these three characteristics will ensure his mastery and continued survival. Their loss will ensure his downfall.

From those savage primitive times down through the Sumerian, Egyptian, Roman and medieval eras, Man has remained basically the same, a unique individual, dangerously aggressive, uncertain of his future, living in complex societies, yet always alone.

Always alone. Most people are aware of it, but never

realize it. You are locked into your body with your thoughts, and everyone else is a stranger with whom to some degree you become acquainted. Even your mother is a stranger to you, for her thoughts and intentions are always unknown to you. True, some communication is possible, but at best it is only a very basic exchange, and forever you will remain a separate individual. The more you feel you have reached rapport and understanding, the more you will deceive yourself.

You were born into the world alone, and so you will remain. Acceptance and integration may blur your appreciation of this fact, but until the hour of your death you will remain unique, alone among the teeming millions of your kind.

If this momentuous circumstance were not sufficient, Man is unique in another frightening understanding. He is the only animal who knows he will die.

So although the mechanics of reproduction and birth are fully understood, every sensible person is positively certain that his individual intelligence, and his personal sense of identity, are something apart and beyond the union of his parents. Equally, and even more, he is satisfied that his identity will not perish into oblivion with his body. Even the most primitive savages, who cannot formulate the thought, know this.

Knowledge of a limited span of life, family obligations and personal desires, allied to rational human aggression, make Man a competitive restless animal actuated by motives of personal gain.

In the earliest days of dynastic Egypt there were men who owned great farms with hundreds of serfs and slaves, who established harems of beautiful women and filled ornate coffers with treasure — but, they could eat only one dinner every day, and they knew that their tenure was fleetingly transient and could only end in a magnificent tomb that would be degraded by time or robbers. Yet they fought and schemed to achieve wealth and rank, and thought any success worth while.

These are the reasons why a utopian, universal peace was never achieved at any time in history, and never will be in the future. A state of perfect equality of ownership and authority cannot exist in this world. Man realizes this and believes, therefore, that it exists in the next world.

Wealthy empires and communities have always needed to fear their poorer neighbours and logical arguments or theological precepts are no defence against invaders. A Chinese sage, when his city was beleaguered by Mongol invaders, went out alone and reproached the attackers for their fury and greed, and offered to help them to lead better lives. The Mongol leader thanked him profusely and explained that their idea of a better life was regular meals — and then they ate him! The moral would seem to be, 'Send a messenger with a note and remain inside the city.'

An eloquent speaker can make most ideas sensible and convincing but he cannot make a theory practical. We all, at some time or another, have altruistic ideas of bettering the lot of humanity, and it is a self-evident fact that those who are most eloquent and respected seem personally to do very well out of it.

So. . . . Man is the aggressive, contumacious, acquisitive, stubborn, assertive, muddle-headed culmination of 3,000 million years of evolution, and you can jolly well be proud of him.

---

3. The Dangers of Self-Diagnosis

It is just not possible, without expert training and considerable experience, to evaluate symptoms correctly and to diagnose disorders accurately. Yet well-meaning, sensible people do it all the time and some are so confident and self-convincing that they terrify themselves.

The commonest type who comes in to see us is usully slightly bowed and walking slowly. Looking at us with apprehensive eyes he (or she) says: 'It's my heart!' Never under any circumstances is it 'my Bell's palsy' or 'my Xerophthalmia'. Just heart; they **know** they have one of those!

Of course there is usually nothing wrong with them at all. Often it is nothing more then just wind under the heart, and easily treated by powdered charcoal in a drink of water.

Nervous tension can give rise to many symptoms that seem to indicate serious disorder and people are often difficult to convince when they think they are right. We call their symptoms pseudo-complaints and seek to treat the underlying causes of their distress, and our case histories abundantly prove that on most occasions we were right.

For example, many women say they have persistent insomnia. This seems to trouble far more women than men. Actually, true insomnia is quite rare and what they suffer from is the result of a psychological inhibition. Simply expressed, this means that they have suffered a period when they had difficulty in sleeping and this has become a fixation and convinced them that they cannot sleep. So now every night when they go to bed the subconscious mind stubbornly insists that they cannot sleep, and no matter how tired and exhausted they are, they stay awake, wretched and miserable.

Of course they all take sleeping pills. One lady inquired if our Nirvana sleeping tablets were effective and Mrs Mitton told her that she was confident that they were. 'Perhaps', replied the lady, after some consideration, 'I had better not take them. I take So-and-So's pills and I can't sleep without them.' Mrs Mitton, interested, asked her how long she had been taking them and whether she took them every night. 'Yes,' answered the lady, 'four every night. I dare not miss them, and I've taken them since 1936.' 'That's 39 years,' said Mrs Mitton and then, rather reasonably I thought, inquired how she knew she could not sleep without them. 'Oh!' was the reply, 'I know I can't,' and that settled that.

The pathetic thing is that she is not unusual. Literally thousands of people throughout this country take pills and tablets every day as a matter of course, confident that they really need them and that they will do them good. Regular assimilation of medication will induce the body to build up an immunity, and when the need really does arise, their essential qualities will have been negatived.

Never take any medication until you are quite certain that you know why you are taking it, and just what you hope to achieve.

If you do not feel well, seek competent advice before you treat yourself. Supposition and personal conviction will often delay essential treatment and perhaps subsequently delay recovery; advice from an amateur or inexpert diagnostician can lead to the same result.

The golden rule with all medication is to take it until you are better and then stop.

---

4. Medical Terms

Alterative	Any substance that can beneficially alter the condition of a patient
Anodyne	Any pain-relieving substance.
Anthelmintic	Any substance causing death and elimination of worms in the body.
Antiseptic	Any substance that prevents putrefaction.
Antispasmodic	Any substance that prevents or relieves spasms.
Aperient	Any substance producing the natural evacuation of the bowels.
Aphrodisiac	Any substance that stimulates sexual functions.
Aromatic	Any substance having a scent or aroma.
Astringent	Any substance that causes contraction of the tissues.
Balsamic	Any substance containing resin or benzoic acid.
Cardiac	Any condition affecting or pertaining to the heart.
Carminative	Any substance that relieves pains caused by flatulence.
Cathartic	Any substance that induces stimulation of bowel action; rather stronger than aperients.
Cholagogue	Any substance that increases the flow of bile.
Corrective	Any substance that restores normal conditions.
Dumulcent	Any substance that soothes and protects the alimentary canal.
Deobstruent	Any substance that frees the natural orifices of the body.
Dermatic	Medication that acts upon the skin.
Diaphoretic	Any drug that induces perspiration.
Digestive	Any substance that aids digestion.

Diuretic	Any substance that increases the flow of urine.
Emetic	Any substance that causes vomiting.
Emmenagogue	Any drug that stimulates menstruation.
Emollient	Any substance that soothes and lubricates.
Expectorant	Any substance that removes matter from the bronchial tubes and promotes expectoration.
Febrifuge	Any substance that reduces feverish conditions.
Haemostatic	Any substance that checks bleeding, aids the clotting of blood.
Hepatic	Any substance that acts upon the liver.
Hydragogue	Any substance that induces the watery evacuation of the bowels.
Hypnotic	Any drug that produces sleep.
Insecticide	Any substance that is fatal to insects.
Laxative	Any substance that induces gentle, easy bowel action.
Mydriatic	Any substance that dilates the pupil of the eye.
Myotic	Any substance that contracts the pupil of the eye.
Narcotic	Any drug that induces stupor and insensibility.
Nephritic	Any drug that affects the kidneys.
Nervine	Any substance that restores the nerves to a normal tone.
Oxytocic	Any drug that contracts the uterus and hastens childbirth.
Parturient	Any product used during childbirth.
Pectoral	Any drug taken orally for chest and lung disorders.
Purgative	Any strong drug that induces evacuation.
Resolvent	Any substance that reduces swelling.
Rubefacient	Any substance that produces inflammation of the skin.
Sedative	Any substance used to placate 'nerves'.
Stimulant	Any substance used to promote the reserve power of the body and produce strength and energy.
Stomachic	Any substance that allays stomach disorders.
Styptic	Any substance that aids the clotting of the blood.
Tonic	Any substance that, if used regularly, will promote vicacity and wellbeing.
Vermifuge	Any substance that expels worms from the body.
Vulnerary	Any substance that promotes the healing of wounds.

5. Ailments and Some of Their Symptoms

Acne	The common acne or adolescent 'spots'. Revealed by a combination of whiteheads, blackheads and red spots prominently displayed, mainly on face, neck and chest. Complexion and hair become greasy.
Acne Rosacea	Persistent flushes and dilation of facial blood vessels, some stomach upsets and often unsightly red pustules on the face. The condition can become permanent.

Acne Variobilormis   A condition in which the skin of the forehead becomes red and irritable.

Adenoids   A swelling at the back of the nose and throat owing to glandular disturbance. Can cause ear troubles and result in frequent colds and throat infections.

Agoraphobia   A psychotic condition in which the sufferer fears wide, open places and hesitates to leave home.

Ague   Feverish chills allied with depression and fatigue.

Alopecia   The word means loss of hair. Bald patches appear on the scalp, usually as a result of emotional upsets or nervous tension.

Amenorrhoea   The cessation of the menstrual flow.

Anaemia   A condition in which there is a deficiency of haemoglobin (red blood cells). It causes exhaustion and swelling of the ankles, and the sufferer exhibits a pale and pallid appearance.

Anal Fissure   A sore or deep groove, or perhaps a breakthrough, in the rectal passage.

Anal Fistula   A chronic condition in which an abscess in the rectal passage has perforated the bowel and allowed excreta to leak out.

Aneurysm   The dilation of an arterial wall. This causes great pain and discomfort. Physical effort must be avoided.

Angina   Fierce pain in the upper chest, neck and left arm are accompanied by a feeling of intense suffocation.

Angina Pectoris   Similar, but pains are spasmodic and the sufferer feels strangled.

Appendicitis   Severe pains in the centre of the abdomen and some sickness. Pain shifts to lower right-hand side of body area. Pressure may reveal a tender spot. Temperature will be increased a little.

Arteriosclerosis   This is a slowly progressive disorder, the effect of hardening and constriction of the arteries.

Arthritis   Revealed by a loss of mobility and stiffness of the joints. Some lumps will appear. Pain varies and can be worse in cold, wet weather.

Asthma   A distressing difficulty in breathing and exhaling. Persistent coughing and wheezing exhaust the sufferer.

Athlete's Foot   A fungus infection between the toes.

Bronchitis   Exhausting bouts of coughing, necessary to clear choking obstructions of mucus, and difficulty in breathing.

Bursitis   A flabby, fluid swelling that is tender and painful. Usually occurs at a joint, most often the knee or elbow.

Chickenpox   Begins as a rash of dark pink spots which quickly blister and become scabs. It starts in the mouth and on the head. Some fever with temperatures up to 102°F.

Cholera   An epidemic disease characterized by severe vomiting and acute diarrhoea.

Cirrhosis	Often a terminal condition, when the liver is hardened and contracted so that its working efficiency is impaired.
Colic	**A sensation of coldness with vomiting. The sufferer is doubled up by agonizing pains.** Flatulence and diarrhoea occur.
Colitis	A severe condition of inflammation of the colon accompanied by fever and blood-stained diarrhoea.
Conjunctivitis	An eye inflammation which usually spreads to both eyes. Some discharge, with irritation and blurred vision.
Cramp	Muscles are locked temporarily with excruciating pain.
Cystitis	Bladder inflammation which necessitates frequent, painful urination.
Dermatitis	An inflammatory skin rash which supurates. It is not contagious and may in some cases be due to industrial contamination.
Diabetes	A disease which inhibits the bodies use of sugar for nutrition due to a lack of insulin.
Diphtheria	A dangerous fever located in the mucous membranes of the throat. It is most highly infectious.
Disseminated Sclerosis	A degenerative deterioration of the nerves of the brain and spinal cord. There is no cure known.
Diverticulitis	Inflammation of the intestine causing pain and diarrhoea.
Dropsy	Originates from several conditions. Can result in the accumulation of fluid in the body, usually at first at the ankles.
Duodenal Ulcer	Ulceration in the duodenum (or other locations in the digestive system, when the prefix will be different) which gives rise to severe flatulence and indigestion causing debility and depression. A serious condition which can respond quickly to treatment.
Dysentry	A bacillary disease responsible for severe diarrhoea and the passing of blood.
Dysemenorrhoea	Excessive pain during menstruation.
Eczema	A red, suppurating skin condition that causes intense irritation. It is very difficult to clear up.
Emphysema	A development of bronchitis in which there is chronic dilation of the lungs. The symptoms are similar to bronchitis but the condition is permanent.
Encephalitis	A condition of brain inflammation due to infection. A most serious disorder.
Fibrositis	Severe muscular pains of a spasmodic nature which restrict mobility.
Gastroenteritis	Inflammation of intestines and stomach which results in severe vomiting and diarrhoea.
German Measles	Shivering and headaches with swollen glands of the neck, followed within a day by pink eruptions which spread all over the body.
Gingivitis	A severe gum infection which can cause bleeding. Very

contagious.

Glandular Fever — Considerable swelling of the glands in the neck, a high fever, and most marked loss of appetite. Very infectious.

Gonorrhoea — **Men:** Severe irritation of the urethra and great pain when urinating. There is a thick yellowish discharge and some swelling in the groin. The urine contains matter with the appearance of threads.
Women: A yellowish discharge from the vagina, severe pains when urinating and inflammation of the glands located in the vulva.

Gout — Severe inflammation of the joints, usually the big toes, caused by excessive amounts of uric acid in the blood. The pain is excruciating.

Gravel — Small stones accreted in the kidneys and bladder which are passed with the urine. The pains are very severe.

Haemorrhoids — Engorged and inflamed veins in the anal passage which give rise to tenderness and pain. Some bleeding when excreting.

Hay Fever — Inflammation of the nose and throat with persistent sneezing. Eyes water frequently and sufferer feels run down.

Hepatitis — An inflammatory infection of the liver which can result in jaundice. Some loss of appetite with sickness and diarrhoea.

Herpes — A virus disorder. Young children will develop swollen glands in the neck, display irritability and become feverish. Adults will develop reddish small swellings on the face or around the genital organs.

Herpes Zoster — Commonly known as shingles. Sufferer becomes feverish and develops a rash with tiny yellow centres. These spread and occasion severe pain. It is a difficult condition to allay.

Hydrocele — Fluid in the testicles due to inflammation. The weight of the fluid causes aching pains in the genitals.

Hypertension — High blood pressure. Some giddiness and headaches at the back of the skull may reveal the condition, which can be serious.

Hypotension — Very low blood pressure. A condition that is often accompanied by physical exhaustion and fainting.

Infantile Paralysis — Some aches and pains and an increase in temperature, often followed by rapid paralysis. An infectious disease.

Influenza — In no way related to the common cold. It is a virus disease that manifests itself by a sudden fever and pains. It can cause severe nosebleeds and physical exhaustion.

Jaundice — A yellowish stain spreads into the whites of the eyes and then slowly discolours the whole skin. Urine is green and dank, tongue furred, and there is a bitter taste in the mouth.

Laryngitis — An inflammation of the larynx causing the loss of the voice and some difficulty in swallowing.

Leucorrhoea — A whitish vaginal discharge often with an offensive odour. Usually associated with conditions of debility.

Lumbago — Spasmodic pains of crippling severity in the lower parts of the back.

Mastitis	An inflamed swelling of the breast which usually occurs during breast-feeding.
Mastoids	The disease of a bone behind the ear. Severe earaches and loss of sleep are the outward manifestations.
Meningitis	The membranes containing the brain become inflamed. The neck is stiffened, and the patient will vomit and suffer from severe headaches. The condition may result in paralysis or coma.
Migraine	Extremely severe headahces, some sickness and the sensation of flashing lights before the eyes.
Mumps	The throat glands before the ear swell up quickly and the sufferer feels low-spirited and debilitated. It is very infectious.
Muscular Dystrophy	A progressive disease that can begin during childhood. The muscles waste away.
Myxoedema	This disease is due to the removal, or failure, of the thyroid gland. Progressive mental and physical deterioration result and the sufferer rapidly puts on weight.
Nephritis	Kidney inflammation. Some fever and pains in the back reveal this condition.
Neuraliga	Agonizing recurrent pain in the face or, rarely, in other parts of the body.
Neuritis	Very severe pains in the sheathes of the nerves which can have a crippling effect for a limited period. Some anxiety and insomnia will occur.
Pancreatitis	Agonizing persistent pains in the stomach due to an inflammation of the pancreas.
Phlebitis	A vein inflammation resulting in the formation of a blood clot. If the clot moves freely the condition can quickly become very dangerous.
Pleurisy	Pains in the side of the chest exacerbated by deep breathing. There is some fever and a most painful cough.
Pneumonia	Shivering, pains in the chest and vomiting. Breathing becomes difficult and temperature rises. Red-brown sputum is expectorated.
Prurigo	A severe skin inflammation which causes small pimples all over the body and continual itching. The sufferer finds it most difficult to rest or to sleep properly.
Psoriasis	A very common and most distressing skin disease. Red, scaly patches appear all over the body and are most difficult to eradicate. The sufferer becomes depressed and anxious.
Pyorrhoea	An infection of the gums giving rise to the discharge of pus. Long continuance can result in the poisoning of the system.
Quinsy	An abscess of the tonsils.
Raynaud's Disease	A nervous disorder which causes the fingers, ears or nose to become white and feel dead. When acute, serious wounds will not bleed.
Rheumatic Fever	Usually affects the young. A severe fever inculcates swelling

of the joints and a weakening of the heart.

Rheumatism   Difficult to define, for so many rheumatoid disorders have individual names. In general, rheumatism can be described as inflammation of the joints with considerable pain and limitations of mobility.

Scarlet Fever   A severe feverish condition with headaches, sore throat and a vivid red rash. Highly contagious.

Stroke   Apoplexy. A gravely severe and often fatal brain condition. Sudden unconsciousness and loss of conscious muscular action is followed by strangled breathing and a slowing of the pulse. The symptoms are very similar to alcoholic drunkenness.

Synovitis   The accumulation of fluid in a joint as the result of an injury. The pain is severe.

Syphilis   Becomes apparent as an almost incurable ulcer on the genitals. The glands become swollen and appetite fails. Some rise in temperature will occur and a faint red rash appears upon the chest. A most serious malady indeed.

Tapeworm   A great increase in appetite will be discernible. There will also be some colic and diarrhoea.

Threadworms   A constant itching of the anal passage with insomnia and nervous tension are the usual symptoms.

Thrombosis   Severe oppressive pains in the chest and a feeble pulse are the first signs. The countenance becomes pallid and breathing shallow. Some vomiting is possible.

Thrush   A fungus infection of the throat. A common condition among weak children.

Tuberculosis   A morning cough of a nervous character with a trifling show of sputum. A loss of appetite and strength will follow and then the sufferer will begin to spit up blood.

Typhoid Fever   Enteric fever. The symptoms are most difficult to discern. Some nosebleeding and night fever will occur.

Typhus   Begins with severe headaches and backaches, some loss of appetite and persistent sickness. Temperature rises rapidly. The rash that follows begins at the wrists and rapidly spreads over the whole body.

Urticaria   Nettle rash. A rash with eruptions of red and white patches which cause great iching.

Varicose Ulcer   The formation of an ulcer on a varicose vein, usually in the leg. Sufferers are mostly advanced in years and the ulcers are very difficult to heal.

Whooping Cough   Some feverishness, watering of the eyes and a cough. The condition develops into paroxysms of coughing and the 'whooping' sound as the sufferer breaths in.

---

6. Diets—Fallacies and Fads

Man has evolved as an omnivorous feeder; that is, he eats a mixed carnivorous and herbivorous diet and thrives on it.

This incontrovertible fact can easily be proved. Stand before a mirror, open your mouth wide, and look carefully at your teeth. You will observe that you have 32 adult teeth, 16 in each jaw, and that they are very obviously intended for different purposes. In each jaw you will have 4 incisors, teeth designed for cutting, 2 canines, teeth designed for wounding and tearing, and 4 premolars and 6 molars, teeth designed for mascerating and grinding. This dental armoury enables Man confidently to eat anything—insects, animals, birds and every kind of vegetation from seeds and fruits to leaves and roots.

When the primitive ancestor of modern man first left the trees and wandered on to the grassy savannas of Africa and Asia, he was vulnerable because he was weaponless and too weak to defend himself from the larger carnivores, and he had left behind the easily gathered foods he was used to. Alertness, agility and speedy flight saved him from the carnivores and his omnivorous, rapacious diet saved him from starvation. He ate everything and anything he could find to eat.

When we were in the Queensland outback we stopped the car to watch a tribe of Australian aborigines pass by, they were, our friend an old Australian outback man told us, the last of a once numerous tribe that was now nearing extinction: there were only twelve of them. The leader was a man with a withered leg who looked old and senile. There were three other men, all of them young and one little more than a boy, and three women with five children, one still at the breast. They were all quite naked. The women carried rough baskets plaited from leaves slung over their shoulders, and the men weapons—the usual stone-tipped spears. Their mode of progression was remarkable, for they were walking in a line abreast with about fifteen feet between each of them and they were bent over intently studying the ground as they went. They kept turning stones over with their hands and feet and frequently snatched at something they had discovered and thrust it, wriggling fiercely, into their mouths.

It's all good tucker,' our friend told us, 'There's no need for anyone to go hungry out here.' We agreed with him and said we did not feel hungry.

When he gave the leader a cigarette and a stale ham sandwich he ate them both and carried on while we put a kettle on to boil. By the time the kettle had boiled and we were making tea they were almost out of sight, and the contact between Stone Age and modern cultures was forgotten.

'They walk about twenty miles a day,' explained our friend when we questioned him, 'and they're making for a water hole. When they get there they'll laze about and eat the water lily roots until they run short and have to move on. Then they'll have to cross the foothills and walk for three days before they come to water again.'

'Can't they settle?' we asked. 'Never,' he told us, 'for they run out of food and have to carry on.' Their territory, he explained, was a dry, arid, near-desert, and it took them about a year to journey around it, forced on by the necessity to find food. Once they had been a strong tribe with witch doctors and many young men to perform their intricate rituals and corroberees, but now the last few were wandering into oblivion. Soon the territory would be empty and the voices of man forever stilled. Perhaps the climate had changed and it was drier than it used to be.

The aborigines reached Australia more than 30,000 years ago during the Ice Age when the sea level was lowered over 300 feet by the vast accumulations of ice in the polar regions. They walked across what are now the islands of Sumatra and Java and arrived in the Northern Territory to find a vast land that had virtually nothing to offer. For Australia, so long cut off from the rest of the world, was a fossilised enclave from the distant past. The highest animals were all primitive marsupial mammals, and there were no plants that man could cultivate, and no fruits that he could plant and harvest. There was nothing besides scenic beauty and solitude.

Never in their history have the aborigines built a hut, for the inexorable necessity to search for sustenance would have made it impossible for them to dwell in it. Nor were there ever any mammals they could domesticate and herd, so they were forced to eat what they could find and were doomed to a perpetual 'walkabout' to search for it. It was widely stated in the early days of colonization that they were Stone Age people and the lowest race of mankind, but study has revealed that, in fact, they are governed by strong social and moral customs and have rigid tribal laws. The aborigine's chance of development to nationhood was hindered by a hostile environment. We observed that they were a perceptive, intelligent people of better than average physique, and were blessed with great endurance and vigour.

Our inquiries revealed that stomach troubles were almost unknown among them and that few exhibited any signs of nervous tension or emotional disorders. Those who did were among the people who lived in settlements upon the white man's bounty. Their natural diet was, of course, to white Australians repulsive, but 30,000 years of it had built the aborigines into a strong and virile people. In every respect their size, strength and endurance equalled the white man's.

We have noted that people we have met in different parts of the world who perforce are vegetarians tend to be of diminutive physique and lacking in strength, and die of old age soon after they are forty! Indian villagers whom we measured in the Punjab averaged about 5ft 1½in in height for men and 4ft 9in for women; but Indians resident in South Africa, the descendants of indentured labourers who came from the Punjab to work in the sugar fields in 1861,

averaged 5ft 6½in for men and 5ft 3 in for women.
Furthermore, fairly accurate statistics showed that the
average life expectancy for men and women in India was
respectively 42 and 45 years. In South Africa it was 54 and
58 years. Religion and social behaviour were precisely the
same but the food differed. The former were vegetarians;
the latter wer able to afford a well-balanced diet.

Man was designed by evolution to eat an omnivorous diet
and, moreover, to **digest** an omnivorous diet. His complete
entition is actually necessary. Vegetarians, with only a
minute number of exceptions, are at a considerable
disadvantage compared with those who enjoy a normal diet.

People who adopt a strict vegetarian diet late in life are at
an especially great risk. We have had many come into our
shop. They usually complain of lassitude and insomnia and
ask for help with digestive troubles. They explain
vociferously that their troubles are due to everything except
the obvious reason—malnutrition. If these people persist in
their decision to live as vegetarians they could become
anaemic, and many of them do so.

Just as the fuel an engine consumes governs its
performance, so the food you eat builds your strength,
vitality and physique. Eat well, and you will stay well. If you
must discriminate, do it against something other than food!

---

7. Some Recommended Diets

Herbal practitioners are required to produce beneficial
results quickly, and for this reason their advice is always
simple, easy and inexpensive to follow — and devoid of
worry complications. It may be considered impressive to
discourse larnedly upon carbohydrates, proteins, fat-soluble
vitamins and calories, but the patient will find them difficult
to understand and remember. Thus the herbalist will
recommended a diet in the simplest possible terms, in a
manner that will be fully understood and can be followed
without doubt and indecision. While the simplicity of
description and usage are deliberate, the intention is always
highly ethical. The long experience and training of a
herbalist are a sufficient guarantee of the value of the
advice.

We cannot stress too strongly the value of consultation. If
you are not sure about a disorder call upon a herbalist or
other specialist, explain your symptoms and ask for advice.

Diet A   To reduce weight quickly and safely

Eat No:	Fat meats, fresh bread, cakes, nuts or sweets or sugar. Use butter or margerine sparingly
Breakfast could be:	1 small plate of breakfast cereal with a little milk plus 1 kipper, **or** 1 rasher of bacon, **or** 1 slice of lean beef or corned beef, and a very thin slice of buttered toast
Mid-morning:	1 cup of weak tea or coffee with 1 dry digestive biscuit

Lunch: a generous slice of corned beef, or lean beef, with salad and tomato

Mid-afternoon: 1 cup of weak tea or coffee with 1 dry digestive biscuit

Dinner: a plate of warm lean beef, or corned beef, with vegetable salad, a baked apple, jelly or fresh fruit

(Instead of lean beef or corned beef you could have grilled kidney, steamed or grilled white fish, roast chicken, a lamb chop with fat removed, or lean ham.)

Lastly, exercise! Walk as much as possible and most certainly have a sharp fifteen minutes walk after turning off the television and before going to bed.

Diet B To increase weight

This is a high-energy, body-building diet that will result in unhealthy flabby fat unless the patient exercises. If the patient is in normal health he or she should have dramatic and successful results in a few weeks.

Breakfast: milk, tea or coffee, made with milk and well sweetened; fried bacon, eggs and tomato with well-buttered bread or toast; marmalade

Mid-morning: milky sweetened tea or coffee with cakes

Lunch: baked beans on toast with a sweet with cream

Mid-afternoon: milky sweetened tea or coffee with cakes

Dinner: a generous helping of any meat dish prepared in any manner with potatoes and vegetables, baked or steamed pudding and cheese and biscuits

A glass of milk stout, or sherry, will help if taken twice a day.

Just because you are underweight, however, you cannot accept all this rich food as a free bonus — you have got to work for it! The apparatus you will require for your exercise is cheap enough though. All you will need is a skipping rope and determination: the former can be much shorter than the latter!

In the morning, take a ten-minute walk after breakfast. During the after noon practise touching your toes with your knees straight for ten minutes, and skip for another ten minutes during the evening. Before retiring walk smartly for at least ten minutes. That is less than an hour's exercise daily, and even if **you** hate it, your body will love it! One word of warning. If you are not used to exercise take things slowly at first and if you begin to feel strained—STOP IMMEDIATELY.

Diet C Diet for sufferers from duodenal ulcers

Eat No: salads or fruit; soups or stews; fried foods; nuts; roast or grilled meats or sausages.

Drink half a glass of tepid water every two hours

Breakfast: 1 cup of tepid, weak Ovaltine (or similar), a little porridge with the top of the milk (best sweetened with honey)

Mid-morning: 1 cup of tepid, weak Ovaltine (or similar) with a sweet biscuit (chew the biscuit as long as possible before swallowing it to promote the flow of the salivary juices)

Lunch: a little warm sweetened milk with a small bowl of Slippery Elm food

Mid-afternoon: 1 cup of tepid weak Ovaltine (or similar) with a sweet biscuit

Dinner: 2 lightly boiled eggs, or steamed or poached white fish, with 1 slice of very thin well-buttered bread

Sit up frequently to bring up the wind and take 2 Cathay charcoal tablets after every meal.

Now to allay the prime cause of the ulcer-nervous tension. Take two Cathay Savant tablets after breakfast, lunch and dinner (that is, six daily). After one week the tension should be so relieved that only four Cathay Savant tablets need to be taken daily, two after breakfast and two after dinner. It will help if two Ginseng Compound tablets are taken each night as well. At the end of the second week the patient should start to improve and thereafter a gradual and steady improvement should be noticeable.

Diet D   For sufferers from rheumatoid disorders

This is simple. Avoid meats, all soups and stews and eat from the following:

Milk, cheese, eggs, fish (not fried), all kinds of poultry, potatoes and fruits. The golden rule is eat little and often, and never have a big meal. It is also helpful to cut the consumption of alcohol drastically.

Diet E   For sufferers from sea-sickness or travel sickness

Paradoxically, one must eat to avoid sea-sickness, for people with empty stomachs are always sick first — and they suffer most. This diet is one that could prove of benefit.

Breakfast: a cup of sweet luke-warm tea with a little well grilled steak and buttered toast

Mid-morning: a cup of tea and two dry biscuits

Lunch: 2 eggs on toast, **or** a lean lamb chop, **or** steak, **no vegetables**

Mid-afternoon: a cup of tea and two dry biscuits

Dinner: Any lean meat with just a little potato, followed by cheese and biscuits

Do not drink alcohol or take too much water. Stay off your bunk and out of your cabin. Get up on deck and keep active. It also helps to have something to take your mind off your worries. Demand to see the captain and complain that his navigation is faulty. You may have to walk the plank but you will not be sea-sick while you are doing it!

8.   How Herbs are Prepared for Use

Methods that are quick and simple to follow.

Infusions The herbs to be used can be fresh or dried, and they may be in the form of seeds, leaves, roots, twigs or flowers. See Part

Two for Parts used of different herbs.

Estimate the quantity of the infusion that you will require, allowing as a general rule about 1 ounce of the herb material to 1 pint of water.

Beat and bruise the material on a chopping block to ensure greater efficacy.

Place the material in an earthenware vessel — a teapot is best. Do not use an aluminium receptacle. Pour 1 pint of boiling water over it. Cover the vessel with heat-retaining material and allow to stand for about thirty minutes. Strain and store the fluid in an airtight bottle. A well-washed fruit drink bottle is excellent. Keep in a cool dark cupboard or on the bottom shelf of a refrigerator. Never make more then is sufficient for 2-3 days.

Dosage. This will differ according to the formulation. Anything between a tablespoonful and a wineglassful taken two to three times daily can be sufficient.

Decoctions

This method is usually used to extract the therapeutic agents from barks and roots where a simple infusion would not prove to be sufficient.

Cut the bark or roots into small pieces about an inch long and beat on a wooden chopping block until they are shredded. Then place about 1 ounce of the material in an iron pot and cover with about 1½ pints of cold water. Boil until about one-third of the water has evaporated. Stand and allow to cool. Strain and store the resulting fluid in a similar manner to an infusion.

Dosage. Varies. In most cases a wineglassful two to three times daily will prove sufficient.

Solid Extracts

This method of preparation simply reduces an infusion, or the fresh juice of herbs, to the consistency of treacle. The material is simmered very gently for a long period, keeping well stirred to prevent burning, until most of the water is boiled off. It should then be stored in an earthenware vessel in a refrigerator and used quickly. Solid extracts are commercially made for the preparation of tablets, pills and ointments. the process they use employs alcohol which is recovered afterwards by distillation.

Methods that necessitate special apparatus

Maceration

The herbs to be used must be crushed and powdered. Place in a clean vessel (not enamelware, aluminium or plastic — an earthenware jug is best) and cover five times the depth of the material with alcoholic menstruum. This is a mixture of 3 parts water to 1 part ALCOHOL. Under no circumstances use wood alcohol. Allow to stand in a cool dark place for twelve hours and then strain off.

Dosage. A teaspoonful three times daily.

Warning. If you know someone who says he can obtain a little alcohol from his place of employment, be careful. The alcohol will probably be wood alcohol, which is a dreadful poison. Alcohol is not generally sold to the public, but a chemist may be able to help you.

Liquid Extracts

These are the most concentrated forms of herbal drugs. They are made to a strength of 1-1; this means that 1 fluid ounce equals 1 ounce of herbs. They keep well and have the great merit of being easy and reliable to use and the dosage can always be exact.

The best method of preparation is to evaporate the alcoholic extraction, made from the herb soaked in a vacuum vessel. The liquid will evaporate until the liquid extract is of the correct volume. Liquid extracts may also be prepared in a pressure vessel or by percolation.

In all cases special equipment will be necessary. This can be obtained from a wholesale chemist who will advise upon the choice of apparatus if told the quantities envisaged.

Tinctures

Many herbal drugs are destroyed by heat and cannot satisfactorily be extracted by water alone. They are best prepared as tincture made with spirits of wine, in which form they persist better and are more efficacious.

Steep the herbs in spirits of wine, about 2 ounces to the pint, in a closed vessel for twelve hours. Strain and bottle. Keep in a cool dark dry place. If the herbs to be used are fresh, bruise them thoroughly before use.

Pills

This is the oldest known method of administering solid medication in predetermined doses. Pills were commonly made in China over 4,000 years ago. The constituents, in extract or crude form, are mixed wet with excipients such as glucose and edible gums, and then rolled in grooves on a board with a smooth piece of wood until they are firm and uniform in size. They are now pearl-coated, but can be rolled in dry icing sugar or powdered liquorice to conceal the noxious taste. Pills are losing in popularity, for they have a shorter shelf life than tablets and clinical purity is more difficult to achieve.

Tablets

The herbal drugs are very thoroughly mixed and then subjected to great mechanical pressure in special compressing machines using stainless steel punches and dies. Various coatings, but mostly sugar, are used to conceal the taste.

Tablets keep better than pills, are easily and accurately formulated and dissolve much more quickly in the stomach. They have revolutionized the medicine industry. It is reliably estimated that one year's production in Great Britain alone exceeds 10,000 million.

Capsules

Uniform-sized gelatine containers are made and filled with oils and other fluid material, then sealed by the application of heat. They are principally used for medication that is unpleasant to take. They are without odour or taste, and thus popular with children.

Suppositories and Pessaries

These are shaped vehicles made from quickly-melting material such as cocoa butter. They are used for the introduction of medication, or nourishment, via the anal passage. When used by women for vaginal insertion they are called pessaries.

A Guide To The Therapeutic Properties Of Herbs

Note. It must be realized that this guide offers no more than the information that a certain herb is well reputed to be efficacious for the conditions referred to. Only those reputed to be the most effective and sure to act are listed. Dosage and methods of preparation are dealt with on later pages.

Some of the herbs are poisonous and not available for general sale. Their names are printed below in **bold type**.

Anodyne	Herbs useful in alleviating pain. **Aconite;** Hops; Jamaican Dogwood; **Poppy**
Anthelmintic	Herbs used to expel worms. Aloes; Male Fern: Wormseed; Wormwood
Antibilious	Herbs used to ease sickness. Balmony; Wild Yam
Antiperiodic	Herbs taken to prevent the recurrence of Asian fevers. **Cinchona; Ephedra;** Feverbush; White Willow
Antiseptic	Herbs that prevent the breakdown of cellular tissues. Abscess Root; Echinacea; Eucalyptus; Golden Seal; Kumarhou; Southernwood
Antispasmodic	Herbs that allay spasmodic conditions. Asafoetida; Chamomile; **Lobelia;** Mistletoe; Pulsatilla; Scullcap; **Stramonium;** Valerian
Aperient	Herbs that promote bowel evacuation. Cascara; Jewelweed; Mulberry; Rhubarb
Aphrodisiac	Herbs that stimulate the libido and sexual organs. Asiatica; Damiana; Ginseng; Hydrocotyle; Muira-Puama; Saw Palmetto; **Yohimbe**
Astringent	Herbs that tighten the tissues. Angostura; Calamus; Golden Rod; Meadowsweet; Oak; Winter's Bark
Bitter	Herbs to promote the appetite. Angostura; Damiana; Feverfew; Gentian; Quassia
Cardiac	Herbs that stimulate the heart. Ailanthus; **American Hellebore;** Cereus; **Foxglove;** Kola; **Lily of the Valle; Strophanthus**
Carminative	Herbs that assist the heart. Angelica; Aniseed; Calamus; Ginger; Peppermint
Cathartic	Herbs that promote quick, strong bowel action. **American Mandrake; Bitter apple;** Black Root; Castor Oil; **Colchicum; Croton;** Hedge Hyssop; Indian Physic; Jalap; Poke Root; Senna; **Squill**
Demulcent	Herbs that lubricate the digestive canals. Arrowroot; Comfrey; Iceland Moss; Irish Moss;

Liquorice; Marshmallow; Slippery Elm

Deobstruent	Herbs that ensure natural evacuation.
	Bladderwrack; Buckbean; Olive; Swamp Milkweed; Wild Carrot
Detergent	Herbs that cleanse and stimulate the skin.
	Balmony; Goa; Golden Seal; Soap Tree; Southernwood; Water Betony
Diaphoretic	Herbs that induce perspiration.
	Buchu; Ipecacuanha; **Jaborandi;** Pennyroyal; Yarrow
Digestive	Herbs that aid digestion.
	Comfrey; Paw-paw; Slippery Elm
Diuretic	Herbs that are helpful in urinary disorders.
	Buchu; Clivers; Couchgrass; Parsley Piert; Pellitory; Stone Root; Uva-Ursi
Emetic	Herbs that compel strong vomiting.
	Ipecacuanha; **Lobelia;** Mustard; Vervain
Emmenagogue	Herbs that promote menstruation.
	Black Hellebore; Life Root; Motherwort; Mugwort; Pennyroyal; Rue; Southernwood
Emolient	Herbs that soften tissues.
	Comfrey; Linseed; Liquorice; Marshmallow; Slippery Elm
Expectorant	Herbs that help to expel phlegm from the bronchial tubes.
	Ipecacuanha; **Lobelia;** Lungwort; Mullein; Pleurisy Root; Squill; **Wild Cherry**
Febrifuge	Herbs that allay fevers.
	Aconite; Avens; Balm; **Gelsemium;** Wormwood; Yarrow
Haemostatic	Herbs that allay bleeding.
	Corn Ergot; Cranesbill; Turmeric
Hepatic	Herbs that stimulate liver action.
	Dodder; Culvers Root; Dandelion; Yellow Toadflax
Hydrogogue	Herbs that can expel surplus water from the tissues and promote urination.
	American Mandrake; Caroba; White Bryony
Hypnotic	Herbs that induce sleep.
	Belladonna; Hemlock; Indian Hemp; Mistletoe; **Poppy; Stramonium**
Insecticide	Herbs that will kill insects.
	Derris Root; Musk Seed; Pyrethrum
Irritant	Herbs that cause irritation of the tissues.
	American Ivy; **Bitter Apple;** Mustard; Poison Oak; Thuja
Laxative	Herbs that promote easy bowel action.
	Buckthorn; Cascara; Dandelion; Linseed; Rhubarb; Senna; Slippery Elm
Mydriatic	Herbs that dilate the pupils of the eyes.
	Belladonna; Stramonium
Myotic	Herbs that contract the pupils of the eyes.
	Calabar Bean; Opium
Nervine	Herbs that allay nervous disorders.
	Avens; Kola; Lady's Slipper; Motherwort; Mistletoe;

Muira Puama; Scullcap; Valerian; Vervain

Parasiticide Herbs that destroy body parasites.
Cocculus Indicus

Parturient Herbs that help during childbirth.
Cotton Root; Squaw Vine

Pectoral Herbs that help when taken for lung disorders.
Blue Mallow; Euphorbia; Hartstongue; Hyssop; Irish Moss; Jujube; Linseed; Lungwort; Mullein; Polypody Root; **Wild Cherry**

Purgative Herbs that cause drastic bowel evacuation.
Aloes; **Bitter Apple;** Jalap

Rubefacient Herbs that when rubbed on the skin produce reddening and irritation.
Black Bryony; Cayenne; **Croton;** Turpentine

Sternutatory Herbs that cause violent sneezing.
Black Pepper; Egyptian Soapwort Root; Soapwort

Stimulant Herbs that promote power and strength.
Ginger; **Jaborandi;** Kola; Mate Tea; Prickly Ash; Poplar; Wintergreen

Styptic Herbs that cause quick clotting of the blood.
Avens; Cranesbill Root; Lady's Mantle

Sudorific Herbs that promote profuse perspiration.
Sarsparilla; Vervain

Vermifuge Herbs that rid the body of worms.
Black Horehound; Blue Cohosh; Goat's Rue; Male Fern; Primrose; Wormseed

Tonic Herbs that promote vivacity and wellbeing.
Damiana; Gentian; Kola; Prickly Ash; Quassia; Unicorn Root

Vulnerary Herbs that cleanse and ensure speedy healing of wounds.
Myrrh; Water Betony

**Effective Herbal Formulae Which Can Be Quickly And Simply Infused
by following the instructions in this chapter**

Ailment	Herbs	Formula (parts)
Acne	Burdock	1
	Blue Flag Root	1
	Clivers	2
	Mate Tea	2
Arthritis	Agrimony	4
	Dandelion	4
	Bogbean	2
	Celery Seed	1
	Burdock	2
Asthma	Iceland Moss	2

	Irish Moss	2
	Ginger	1
	Liquorice	4
	Damiana	2
Back and kidney complaints	Buchu	1
	Wild Carrot	1
	Couchgrass	2
	Horsetail	2
	Nettles	4
	Juniper	1
Bronchitis	Liquorice	8
	Irish Moss	4
	Eucalyptus	2
	Wild Cherry	2
	Marshmallow	8
	Aniseed	1
Cataracts	Eyebright	6
	Golden Seal Root	1
Catarrh	Coltsfoot	4
	Fennel	2
	Vervain	1
	Peppermint	2
Colitis	Fenugreek	8
	Slippery Elm Bark	1
	Comfrey Root	1
Constipation	Senna	4
	Liquorice	2
	Elder Flowers	1
	Fennel Seed	1
Coughs	Horehound	1
	Hyssop	2
	Coltsfoot	2
	Marshmallow	2
	Peppermint	1
	Liquorice	1
Cramp	Avena Sativa	4
	Ginger	1
	Motherwort	2
	Scullcap	1
	Cramp Bark	1
Cystitis	Horsetail	2
	Clivers	2
	Buchu	1
	Broom	2
	Marshmallow	4
Dermatitis	Scullap	1
	Valerian	1
	Mistletoe	2

	Comfrey Leaves	4
Diverticulitis	Marshmallow Root	4
	Fenugreek Seed	8
	Slippery Elm Bark	8
	Ginger	1
Duodenal, or peptic, ulcers	Comfrey	4
	Marshmallow	8
	Slippery Elm	8
	Golden Seal	2
	Poke Root	1
Gastritis	Slippery Elm	4
	Marshmallow	6
	Yarrow	4
	Golden Seal Root	1
Gastroenteritis	Arrowroot	8
	Paprika	2
	Cinnamon	1
Goitre	Fucus Vesiculata	8
	Irish Moss	2
	Marjoram	1
Gout	Couchgrass	2
	Broom	1
	Parsley Leaves	2
	Mate Tea	4
Headache and migraine	Rosemary	1
	Scullcap	1
	Wild Lettuce	1
	Valerian	1
	Balm	2
Hypertension (high blood pressure)	Lily of the Valley	1
	Cactus Flowers	1
	Hawthorn Berries	2
	Nettles	2
Hypotension (low blood pressure)	Lime Tree Flowers	2
	Motherwort	2
	Paprika	1
	Hawthorn Berries	3
Indigestion and flatulence	Gentian	1
	Calamus	2
	Buckthorn	1
	Peppermint	2
	Chamomile	2
Influenza	Holy Thistle	1
	Meadowsweet	1
	Yarrow	2
	Elder Flowers	2
	Peppermint	1

Insomnia	Passiflora	2
	Hops	1
	Wild Lettuce	1
	Lime Tree Flowers	2
Lack of virility	Kola	2
	Damiana	3
	Muira Puama	1
Laryngitis	Thyme	2
	Iceland Moss	4
	Dill	1
	Cassia Bark	1
	Nettles	4
Lumbago	Dandelion Root	4
	Blue Flag Root	1
	Yarrow	4
	Meadowsweet	2
Meniere's Disease	Ginseng	2
	Bayberry	1
	Kola	8
	Mistletoe	4
Nervous tension	Humulus	1
	Mistletoe	3
	Wild Lettuce	2
	Passiflora	2
	Hawthorn	2
	Scullcap	1
	Motherwort	2
	Fucus	4
Neuritis	Jamaican Dogwood	1
	Humulus	3
	Scullcap	1
	Chamomile	2
Obesity	Fucus	8
	Prickly Ash	1
	Calamus	1
	Horsetail	2
	Damiana	2
Piles and haemorrhoids	Pilewort	3
	Stone Root	1
	Dandelion Root	2
	Witch Hazel Bark	1
Pruritis	Kola	4
	Poplar Bark	2
	Gentian	1
	Paprika	1
	Damiana	4
Psoriasis	Wild Lettuce	2
	Passiflora	4

	Mistletoe	2
	Motherwort	4
	Burdock	1
Rheumatism	Cascara	2
	Blue Flag Root	6
	Prickly Ash	2
	Ginger	1
	White Willow Bark	2
Shingles	Hops	2
	Mistletoe	1
	Wild Lettuce	1
	Scullcap	1
	Damiana	1
	Nettles	2
Stones	Clivers	1
	Parsley Piert	2
	Horsetail	1
	Couchgrass	1
	Hydrangea Root	1
Ulcers	Comfrey Leaves	4
	Nettles	4
	Burdock	2
	Dandelion Leaves	2
	Echinacea	1
Varicose veins	Nettles	2
	Motherwort	2
	Hawthorn Berries	1
	Rose Hips	1

9. Equivalent Weights and Measures

Home dispensing equivalents

1 drop	1 minim
1 teaspoon	60 minims (or 1 fluid drachm)
1 dessertspoon	120 minims (or 2 fluid drachms or ¼ oz)
1 tablespoon	½ fluid ounce
Wine glass	2½ fluid ounces
Teacup	5 fluid ounces
Teacup (large)	8 fluid ounces
Glass	10 fluid ounces
1 litre	35.2 fluid ounces
1 decilitre	3.5 fluid ounces
60 minims	1 fluid drachm
8 fluid drachms	1 fluid ounce
20 fluid ounces	1 pint

Temperature conversions

Fahrenheit	Centigrade
0°	−18°
12°	−11°
32°	0°
48°	9°
60°	16°
72°	22°

Miscellaneous equivalents

1 pint	0.59 litres
1 litre	1.76 pints
1 gallon	4.54 litres
5 gallons	22.73 litres
1 kilogram	2.2 pounds
1 mile	1.61 kilometres
1 metre	1.09 yards

Avoirdupos

1 drachm	27.3 grains
16 drachms	1 ounce or 437.5 grains
16 ounces	1 pound
1 pound	453.6 grams

Apothecaries' weights

20 grains	1 scruple
3 scruples	1 drachm
8 drachms	1 ounce

10. What a Well-Stocked Medicine Cabinet Should Contain

1 large tin of assorted adhesive plasters
1 roll of wide plaster strip
gauze dressings
cotton wool
safety pins
tweezers (broad-ended) for removing splinters
eye bath
antiseptic balm
insect repellent
pain relief tablets
travel sickness tablets
charcoal digestive tablets
laxative pills

herbal nerve tranquillizers
liniment embrocation

Note: Always keep medication in a cool, dark, dry place.

---

11.   Suggested Herbal Medication

> The formulae given in this section are suggested for the
> simple reason that, in the light of their very considerable
> experience, the authors know of nothing safer or more
> surely effective.

Asthma

Just as bronchitis is known as the Englishman's Disease, so
asthma is known in the Antipodes as the Australian
Handicap. The reference is derived from horse racing and it
is remarkably accurate, for it is always an odds-against
event and only the non-participants can win.

'Asthma' means 'grasping for breath', which is a very apt
and proper description. Sufferers do indeed gasp for
breath, until they are physically and mentally exhausted.

The incidence of asthma is so high in Australia that from
the very earliest settlement days science has looked for the
cause and cure. It is generally supposed that the long
periods of hot dry weather and dusty atmospheric conditions
are responsible. However, some people claim that allergies
or pollens are the cause, and a few believe that cats and dogs
or some foodstuffs initiate it. They could be right, but
nothing has ever been proven and asthma is still one of the
most prevalent disorders. There are nostrums and
treatments beyond count but none that are totally effective.

When we first went to Australia, we were surprised to
learn that acute sufferers were advised to smoke
stramonium (Datura stramonium), or tobacco, at short
intervals to obtain relief. It seemed like jumping off a high
cliff to cure hiccoughs. We treated the patients who came to
us by attempting to relieve the paroxysms and soothe the the
the bronchial tubes.

Long experience has taught us that some nervous tension
shock can bring about an attack of asthma, and we attempt
to tranquillize a patient and supply a quick emollient
combined with an effective expectorant.

The formula that we use is (per tablet):

Lobelia	90mg
Gum Ammon	
Cayenne	
Liquorice of each	30mg
and the aqueous extractive from	
Scillae	30mg

Its success greatly exceed all our expectations. It provided very quick relief, did not impair mental capabilities and was without any observable side effects.

It can be taken by children over the age of ten years, and by women and men of any age.

Heart, liver and kidney troubles

We do not advise sufferers from serious disorders affecting these organs to treat themselves, or others, at home. We formulate and prepare tonics and toning compounds, but wish to re-iterate that persons should not attempt to diagnose their own maladies, but should consult a doctor.

Bronchitis

This is a distressing condition that occurs when the bronchial tubes are inflamed. It is known in two forms, acute bronchitis and chronic bronchitis. The former is exhausting and debilitating and can become serious if it does not yield to treatment in two weeks. The latter is the well-known bane of old people; it is aggravated by adverse weather, when they should remain sheltered in the warm as much as possible. It causes shortage of breath after slight exertion, and physical exhaustion. If neglected the conditon can become terminal.

Bronchitis is not something similar to a sore throat or a bad cold. It is a serious condition and must be treated as such. Because of possible complications we invariably recommend that all young children suffering from acute bronchitis be treated by a doctor.

We also strongly advise sufferers not to smoke. The sensible will not, anyway, and the others will realize why they should not every time they light a cigarette!

Sufferers should stay in the warm and rest as much as possible. They should eat sparingly and avoid foods that can cause flatulence.

The formula for a helpful tablet that is soothing and has expectorant qualities is as follows (per tablet):

Lobelia	60mg
Ammoniacum	30mg
Cayenne	10mg
Capsicine BPC'23	10mg
and the aqueous extractive from	
Squil	30mg

Catarrh

No named disorder has ever had such nonsense written, or talked, about it than catarrh. Its ramifications seem to be approaching the infinite. People claim to have: nasal catarrh, throat catarrh, chest catarrh, stomach catarrh, rectal catarrh, aural catarrh and many other forms of the disorder.

In fact, catarrh is the name loosely used to describe any irritation of the mucous membrane. This causes heavy mucous secretions which must be expectorated or swallowed.

Heavy smokers will find that catarrh will induce prolific

watery discharge from the nostrils and cause bouts of violent sneezing. The remedy is simple — stop smoking!

In our experience it is a condition that is easily cleared, provided that it does not indicate the presence of bronchial troubles. We produced a simple herbal remedy for it very many years ago. We used some herbs imported from the Far East, made up a batch of 5gr tablets, and prepared to think no more of it. People who tried them, however, particularly older people, were so enthusiastic in their recommendations that the demand grew like a forest fire and we now have to make half a million at a time. We send them to most countries in the world and receive enthusiastic reports of their efficacy almost every day. While we were on a cruise last year, a fellow passenger earnestly recommended Mrs Mitton to take them!

Here is the formula (per tablet):

Lobelia	60mg
Ammoniacum	30mg
Cayenne	10mg
Capscine BPC'23	10mg
and the aqueous extractive from	
Squill	30mg

Their action is very swift and catarrhal conditions are usually abated in a few days.

Constipation

All civilizations and in particular the Romans have been obsessed with constipation. The Romans actually had shops that sold nothing but purgatives and laxatives, and when the new magnificent Roman baths were built by Augustus in Carthage a free enema was offered as an inducement to buy a season ticket.

The evacuation of the bowels is a natural and automatic action and most people have established a rhythm that ensures a satisfactory performance of the function. It is quite unnessary to take purgatives — indeed, if taken regularly they may prove harmful. **Under no circumstances whatever should persons suffering from stomach ulcers take them.**

People think that they should take laxatives to cleanse the system and stay healthy, and many take them regularly without realizing that they do not need them.

The golden rule of health is never to take any medication until you are positive that you really need it. We advise that nothing be taken to relieve constipation until it has persisted for more than four days. Lapses of up to five days are fairly normal and no harm should result. The normal rhythm will then be resumed. If some help is considered necessary, only the mildest laxative should be taken.

Habits differ from country to country. Here in England the demand is for gentle laxatives, whereas in Africa, where people evacuate after every meal, we can sell only very strong purgatives.

Of course, the pattern of life is changing. People are eating richer foods and walking less. They spend more time sitting in overheated rooms watching television, and manual labour is less common. Primitive man evolved as a dominant being because he was an agile, active, curious predator. These qualities are becoming alien to our way of life and perhaps this is one reason for the growing number of sufferers from constipation.

The daily intake of food should be balanced between roughage (that is, bulky low-protein food that will fill the bowel and ensure muscular performance) and high-protein food. It is not possible to digest the latter adequately without eating sufficiently of the former. We advise everyone to eat a generous plateful of breakfast cereal every morning. For most persons, that should take care of any constipation problems.

We have a laxative herbal formula (it is, by the way, recommended for children over the age of eight) which is also put up in tablet form, as follows (per tablet):

Aloe	45mg
Rhei	45mg
Cayenne	33.75mg
Gamboge	10mg
Oil Peppermint	0.0005ml
and the aqueous extractive from	
Cascara	90mg
Jamaica Dogwood	30mg

Duodenal Ulcers*

The ulcers are located in the mucous membrane, the lining of the stomach or the duodenum, and give rise to conditions debility, spasmodic pains and chronic gastritis. They are also one of the most frequent causes of weak virility and impotency. If not relieved they may cause severe malnutrition and anaemia. Stomach ulcers are found more commonly in men than in women. The occurrence of the disorder is so frequent among people with executive responsibility that it is almost regarded as an occupational hazard, and men come to regard it as normal. Nevertheless, it is agonizing, distressing and dangerous, and can result in early death.

We believe that ulcers are the result of an inbalance of the digestive fluids. When food enters the mouth, saliva is exuded from the salivary glands and becomes mixed by the act of chewing. When swallowed the mixture enters the stomach where the gastric juices begin the process of digestion. There is contained in the gastric juices a proportion of free hydrochloric acid, and we believe that when too much is exuded into the stomach it attacks the mucous membrane as well as assisting the natural digestive processes. Gas released by the breakdown of sections of the

*Also gastric ulcers and peptic ulcers.

mucous membrane will give rise to gastritis (inflammation of the stomach) and will result in painful flatulence. Persistence of the imbalance will result in ulcers.

In accordance with our belief in treating the root cause of a persistent ailment rather than the symptoms, we have an analysis of cases which persuades us that acute nervous tension can be a main factor in the imbalance.

Our treatments have been designed to relieve the tension and thus allow nature to restore natural digestion. The results have often been dramatic. A high proportion of sufferers have reported almost complete recovery and the resumption of a normal diet. Many cases in which an operation had been advised were included. In most of these cases the recovery was accomplished in a relatively short time and many who had lived on a diet for years, now eat fried foods without any after-effects. The increase in weight and energy was most marked.

A high proportion of the sufferers were commuters, or who had an onerous and/or monotonous job, or great responsibilities. There were very few labourers or persons with low IQs. So it seems to us that intelligent people who accept a burden of decision are exceptionally susceptible to serious stomach disorder. A suitable diet would be 'diet C' — under the section — Recommended Diets.

The patient should NOT use mustard, salt, pepper or sauces drink carbonated liquids, wines, spirits, beer, exercise or smoke heavily, eat salads, soups, stews or casseroles

The patient should rest for at least half an hour after each meal and drink plenty of water

The herbal medication we recommended is in tablet form.

	Tablet (1)
Motherwort	45mg
Kelp	45mg
Hops	15mg
Aneurin Hyd.	0.3mg
Riboflavin	0.5mg
Nicotinamide	2.5mg

and the aqueous extractive from:
Mistletoe
Wild Lettuce
Passiflora   — of each of these 90mg.
Hawthorn
Scullcap

	Tablet (2)
Slippery Elm	400mg
Oil Cinnamon	
Oil Clove	of each 0.001ml
Oil Peppermint	

Patients are usually able to eat more normal meals within a few weeks.

Gout

Sufferers from gout are usually regarded as figures of comedy, and the disorder is thought to be the result of rich and profligate living. A politician of the last century said: 'A beggar with bronchitis arouses sympathy; a bishop with gout — satisfaction.' But these suppositions are quite fallacious. It is an excruciatingly painful disorder, and the sufferer is rendered helpless.

Gout is reasonably supposed to be hereditary, and the sufferers are usually engaged in sedentary occupations. Few manual workers are troubled by it. It occurs in severely inflamed joints, where there are considerable deposits of urate of soda, and is mostly confined to men past middle age. The very few women who contract it are usually undergoing the menopause. It is most often experienced in the feet, particularly in the big toes, although it can affect the hands.

Absolute rest is quite essential, and the patient should drink tepid water copiously. Diet is important; the patient should eat a high-protein diet, little and often, and eschew rich foods, soups, stews, salads or fruit. He must also abstain from any form of alcohol.

The best known, and the oldest, of all treatments is colchicum (Colchicum autumnale). This is the plant known to most as meadow saffron. Although most effective in its relieving action, it should be used with care, for a little more than the correctly estimated dosage can give rise to violent purging.

We prefer the old American remedy known as Shanghai Pearls. This is just as efficient and far safer to use. We find that in most cases it can give rise to an astonishing improvement in a short time. Each tablet contains:

Sod Salicyl	60mg
Oil Celery	0.001ml
and the aqueous extractive from	
Celery	270mg

Insomnia

The herbalist is always interested in the patient, and if the opportunity arises will seek by question to elicit the cause of the symptoms described. We have been closely interested in the problems of insomnia for very many years, and Mrs Mitton has paid particular attention to its incidence among women. Our conclusions, when thoroughly formulated, surprised us.

We realized that most sufferers were the victims of a psychological inhibition occasioned by 'nerves' which prevented them from sleeping naturally. So the name 'insomnia' in the majority of cases meant the inability to sleep satisfactorily and nothing more. This is a very common condition indeed, and the effects are very disturbing in the long term. Mental exhaustion and confusion become evident and the sufferer is tried, irritable and incompetent.

The cure is basically simple. To begin with, restrict caffeine intake by drinking less tea and coffee. Do not eat a rich and heavy meal shortly before retiring to bed. Make sure that the bed is sufficiently warm to keep the back and feet at an equable temperature, but that it is not too warm to be comfortable. Relieve uncomfortable stomach wind (flatulence) by taking charcoal tablets before retiring.

And last, and most important of all, convince yourself that you will fall asleep and rest undisturbed.

Most insomniacs talk about their insomnia as if it were inevitable and something ordained by the Almighty. They say with conviction 'I never sleep' and because they are absolutely convinced of it, they do not sleep. Their subsconscious mind prompts them and when they are dozing off they come fully awake, frustrated and distressed. If they can break this pattern they will quickly re-establish the rhythm of natural sleep again.

Naturally they need a little help. Mrs Mitton realized this and the medication she suggests is in tablet form and acts to placate tensions and wipe out the subconscious fixation. Its effect is gentle and soothing and it really does induce natural, healthy sleep. Best of all, it is entirely harmless. Each tablet contains:

Vevain	60mg
Lupulus	30mg
and the aqueous extractive from	
Passiflora	of each 90mg
Wild Lettuce	
Valerian	180mg

Lumbago

Lumbago is one of the most common winter disorders. We regard it as a form of rheumatism, characterized by inflammatory conditions of the muscle tissue. It usually manifests itself in the lumbar region of the back and seems to result from a strain, or the after-effects of cold and damp. The pain is excruciating and movements greatly aggravate the agony. Sufferers are hardly able to rise or dress themselves.

We do not need to recommend rest — a bout of lumbago renders that an absolute necessity! In the light of our experience the best remedial treatment is a very gentle massage with a herbal ointment and repeated hot fomentations.

We also recommend the following formula (in tablets):

Burdock	
Yarrow	
Bogbean	of each 30mg
Agrimony	
Raspberry Fol.	
Pot. Tart Acid	
Guaiacum Resin	of each 15mg
Nutmeg	
Sulphur Sub	120mg

Migraine and Headaches

The causes of these very common distressing disorders are not fully understood although some medical authorities ascribe them to dilation of the blood vessels of the brain. Migraine appears to be more common among women than men, and is characterized by sickness and uneasiness preceding the head pains. Patients often say that they are troubled by intense visual impressions of light.

The usually accepted herbal methods of treatment are regular bowel evacuation, with rest and freedom from disturbance or worry. Meals should always be light and easily digested, and we advise sufferers to avoid anything that may disturb digestion, such as raw fruits and vegetables. It helps to practise deep breathing at regular intervals throughout the day.

A patient once told us that chewing gum steadily was a great help during attacks. She said it eased the violent pains quickly, and stopped the sickness.

We recommend herbal nerve tablets to be taken with weak but hot sweet tea, during attacks. The sufferer should then lie down in a darkened room for an hour. Each tablet contains:

Scullcap	45mg
Lupulus	45mg
Gum Asafoetida	30mg
and the aqueous extractive from	
Gentian	85mg
Valerian	100mg

Nervous Tension

It is extraordinary how changes in one's environment and the patterns of life can give rise to what must be regarded as serious health problems. In the many years we have been practising herbalists, it has become more and more apparent to us that nervous tension is becoming a veritable scourge to the populace.

Years ago it was comparatively uncommon. People seemed to accept their lot in life and adjust naturally. Now it is reasonable to suppose that one person in every five is to some degree a sufferer.

The name is innocuous. To say a person suffers from nervous tension conveys the impression that it is nothing more serious than the common cold. Nothing could be further from the truth. Nervous tension can make a person's life almost unbearable, impair marriage and family associations, and ruin careers. In its early stages it will manifest itself by bouts of sudden irritation and resentment, loss of confidence and fits of depression. The young can develop as side-effects eczema or psoriasis, can become withdrawn, or exhibit an inferiority complex. This latter condition may be considered to be shyness or, if accompanied by truculence when questioned, as boorish indifference.

Loneliness

One very common cause of nervous tension is loneliness. This problem is compounded by the fact that so few people are willing to admit that they **are** lonely.

As people grow older, it is quite natural that they should grow away from their early friends. Marriage brings new obligations and objectives, and for a time friends often become less important as contact is less frequent and mutual interests wane. Then, inevitably, the children grow up and leave home, and the house is left quiet and seemingly without a purpose.

This is all in the natural order of things, and loneliness that arises out of it cannot be dealt with by attempting to maintain the old relationship with children who have married and established their own homes. When family obligations and ties have lessened, the time has come to seek new interests and friends.

The possibility of establishing friendships through chance encounters is unfortunately very remote. It is more worth while to join, for example, a political party and volunteer for committee work or the collection of subscriptions. In this way anyone can soon become part of an affable, like-minded association of people in his or her own area. Churches, too, need voluntary helpers, for there are many lonely and sick people who would welcome visits.

No one is alone in his loneliness. Many long for companionship but try to conceal their solitude. By making it your objective to help others, you will be helping yourself.

Some case histories

In order to demonstrate the wide variety of symptoms that nervous tension may give rise to, some examples from our case histories are included.

Mr J.W.M.

Aged 41 years. Married with two children. Employed as a commerical traveller and enjoying comparative financial security. Has recently been promoted to area manager. Complains that he is sleeping poorly and does not arise refreshed. Is troubled by stomach pains after meals and has a lot of flatulence. Suffers bouts of extreme irritability when driving and complains of his neighbours' noisy children and radio. Some rheumatic pains at irregular intervals, and hair is receding and dry. Is worried about his failing virility.

Mrs J.S.

Aged 36. Married with one son. Employed as a cashier. She complains of persistent headaches and insomnia. Is depressed and has fits of crying. Some flatulence and indigestion. Periods irregular with some incidence of menorrhagia. Feels 'run down' and lacks energy. Cannot sit down and rest in the evening, says 'there is always so much to do'. Does not eat breakfast but takes up to six much advertised patent medicine tablets a day.

Miss V.E.

Aged 18. A student. Will shortly take a driving test. Does not eat breakfast, but eats salads every day. Complains of severe migraine and frequent stomach cramps. Is troubled by frequent diarrhoea and heavy periods. Is shy and hesitates to meet strangers. Worries about imminent examinations and lacks confidence. Her hair is dry and dull and her complexion impaired by acne. Has some psoriasis on the upper arms.

Miss I.C. Aged 56. A schoolmistress. Adopted a vegetarian diet five years previously. Is underweight and debilitated. Complains of severe migraine and rheumatic pains which are not static but appear in different parts of her body. Feels very worried and depressed. Unhappy in her flat and troubled by noise, wants to move to a quiet country place. Does not go out much and has few intimate friends. Is an insomniac and regularly takes sleeping pills. Has been under the care of her doctor for many years.

Mr R.W. Aged 52. Employed on a computer. Married with three grown children. Has a duodenal ulcer and lives on a rigid diet. Frequently quarrels with his children, usually over noisy radios. Is irritable and has fits of rage, feels very depressed and sleeps badly. Is afflicted with long-standing psoriasis and is impotent.

These unhappy people were all, in our opinion, suffering from nervous tension, and this was the root cause of all their symptoms. They were people of above-average intelligence and perhaps for that reason accepted a greater degree of personal responsibility for the conduct of their affairs. They are worried deeply about their own and their family's prospects and, sleeping or waking, were unable to divorce themselves from the problem. In short, they were trying to maintain twenty-four hours of conscious mental consideration every day, and the strain was breaking them down.

Ideally, at the end of a frustrating and difficult day a person should be able to forget it completely and enjoy some recreational interests, or just to rest. We all have two minds, the conscious and the subconscious. The former controls directed mental processes arising from external stimuli and animal behaviour, and the latter is responsible for the uncontrolled exploratory thought patterns when the body is quiescent during sleep. The level of mental activity is so high when a person is severely tensed that the sufferer's mind will continue to strive to elucidate an infinity of probabilities when it should be at a low-energy output level of rest.

It was this nagging overload of inconsequential worrying that has dragged the patients we refer to into their miserable conditions of nervous debility and distressing confusion. They were suffering needlessly, and if intelligent considerations and evaluations were necessary they were too tired and confused to provide them.

Countless doctor's prescriptions are written every year for

medicine to alleviate the symptoms instead of eliminating the root cause, and many operations are carried out for the same reason. Of course, a high proportion of the adult population swallow millions of pills and tablets because their objective reasoning is just as faulty.

To repeat what we have said before, herbalists try to seek and understand the prime cause of the symptoms made known to them and to correct that rather than the symptoms themselves. Thus successful treatment can ensure the termination of all the symptoms.

We decided that it would be helpful for the people whose case histories we have reported to go on to a high-protein diet — not a rigorous or irksome diet, but one that would be easy and pleasant to follow. We set it out herewith:

Breakfast

one or two small slices of thin bread and butter, one or two eggs, **or** boiled fish, **or** a slice of corned beef, **or** a rasher of grilled bacon, a small bowl of breakfast cereal with the top of the milk

Mid-morning

a cup of weak tea or cocoa with two digestive biscuits

Lunch

tea, or cocoa, with two small thin well-buttered sandwiches containing lean beef, corned beef, or ham

Mid-afternoon

as mid-morning

Dinner

Beef **or** fish with one potato and a little gravy

They were informed that they could eat as much lean beef or fish as they wished, **but no** soups, casseroles or stews; **No** salads or fruit; if they felt drink was essential then only a glass or two of oatmeal stout. Last, they were to drink plenty of water.

Since it is a sheer waste of time to tell a person suffering from nervous tension to 'stop worrying', we prescribed the medication that we knew by long experience to be quickly effective and without any deleterious side-or after-effects. This formula is made up into tablets, each tablet containing:

Motherwort	45mg
Kelp	45mg
Hops	15mg
Aneurin Hyd.	0.3mg
Riboflavin	0.5
Nicotinamide	2.5mg

and the aqueous extractive from

Mistletoe	90mg

Wild Lettuce	
Passiflora	of each 45mg
Hawthorn	
Scullcap	

We consider these tablets to be as strong and more effective than many tranquillizers, and without the risk of becoming dependent on them.

For the first week we recommended that six tablets should be taken — two each after breakfast, lunch and dinner. After the first week we knew they would feel so relaxed and improved that they could reduce the dose to four tablets daily.

The herb upon which we place the greatest reliance for the alleviation of nervous tension and nervous debility is ginseng (**Panax quinquefolium**). This is the oldest known medicinal herb in the world. It is reported in a manuscript discovered in China dating to 2500 BC. Its therapeutic qualities are not yet fully understood, but it is well known to herbal science and is without question one of the finest nerve stimulants known. It is also a restorative and tonic, and one of the very safest aphrodisiacs for the elderly. To be effective it must be grown wild, above the snow line, and the demand is so great that it is now the costliest medicinal herb in the world. A little is always insufficient, for it is very slow to manifest its therapeutic powers. To offset this drawback the benefits continue long after it ceases to be taken.

We always recommend that patients should take a full six months' course of two tablets daily, and that is what we recommended our case history people to do.

In addition, we recommended Mrs J.S. and Miss I.C. to take a fluid stimulant, and Miss V.E. and Mr R.W. to use a herbal psoriasis ointment. We asked each of them to report upon their progress at fortnightly intervals, for six weeks. After two reports:

Mr J.W.M. said that his stomach troubles had cleared up and that he was sleeping better; he felt much less tensed and was now coping normally.

Mrs. J.S. said she was feeling very much better and was able to rest. Her family life was much improved.

Miss V.E. reported that her psoriasis had cleared up. She felt relaxed and more confident, and was not so shy.

Miss I.C. reported no discernable improvements.

Mr R.W. was obviously much more relaxed and stomach troubles less evident. However, he still felt his employment to be intolerable.

(Since Mr R.W. consulted us, three or four other computer operators have sought our help. This employment would seem to be exceptionally onerous.)

In general we would advise people who feel they may be 'overtensed' to adopt a hobby that requires high concentration so that they may break the pattern of oppressive inconsequential conjecture. It helps to join a library and make close study of, say, Egyptology or astronomy, or to try to write a novel or short stories, or to draw. Anything that requires close mental attention and breaks the sequences of degenerate thought will do admirably.

A sufferer will be helping to expedite a severe nervous breakdown if he gives in to a desire to sit quietly and feel miserable. He must divert his mental activities into logical processes and sensible appraisals. He must control his intelligence and mental activities, or these will control him!

Herbal medication for the relief of nervous tension and strain is neither hypnotic, narcotic nor soporific. It is at once a nervine, sedative and stimulant, eliminated by the body within forty-eight hours and quite without any side-or after-effects of any kind. In short, it is strongly effective, entirely natural and perfectly wholesome. Sufferers in their own best interests should ensure that any medication they are offered possesses these qualities.

Piles and Haemorrhoids

This is a painful and worrying condition caused by varicose veins either at the terminal end of the anal passage or within the rectum. It is usually due to strain or constipation and is common to many middle-aged people and women during pregnancy.

Severe inflammation will cause the piles to bleed. Copious discharge of blackish blood indicates that the piles are located within the lower bowel.

Sufferers should eat a light, easily digested diet and refrain from violent exercise. Rest is always helpful.

We recommended that a special herbal ointment be gently applied with the tip of a finger in order to reduce and relieve the pile.

We also recommend the following tablet to be used in conjunction with the ointment. The tablets each contain:

Senna fol.	30mg
Pilewort	30mg
and the aqueous extractive from	
Cascara	180mg
Hamamelidis	240mg

Psoriasis

This is a chronic skin disease identified by the ugly, red, scaly eruptions which can spread all over the body and scalp. It is debilitating and also a source of acute embarrassment. It is not contagious, although sufferers should not engage in retail food sales.

Psoriasis is very difficult to eradicate and can persist with varying intensity for many years. It does not generally respond to orthodox medical treatment. Herbal medication, however, can often relieve it effectively and quickly. Our own herbal course regularly produces testimonials from patients who have benefited from it. This course, which we have perfected after treating many hundreds of cases over a long period of years, has the great merit of being simple to use and non-odorous, and the reocurrence of outbreaks is considerably diminished.

Rheumatoid Arthritis And Osteoarthritis

Although adequately named and well known, the causes of these two afflictions are still unknown. It is not even certain that they are variations of the same disease. All that is certain is that they are crippling diseases which kill young and old and that the incidence of them is quickly increasing. The percentage of the population that suffers from one of other grows every year. The distinguishing features are:

Osteoarthritis

A deterioration of the bone structure and enlargement of the joints by calcium deposits. Excruciating pain is usual. When the condition progresses, ankylosis (the permanent locking of joints) occurs and the sufferer is permanently crippled and incapacitated.

Rheumatoid arthritis

This begins with inflammation of the membranes and tissues in the smaller joints and gives rise to extensive deformities which can become permanent. Agonizing pains are usual and often result in loss of confidence, debility and depression.

We have believed for many years that these conditions may be due to a nervous imbalance which starts a chain reaction giving rise to arthritis. Although we have no scientific evidence to support this theory, there are no other feasible theories that disprove it.

When we lived in the Far East we met a lecturer from Hong Kong University who was kind enough to translate some old Chinese medical treatises for us, and one especially aroused our interest. In brief, it said: 'Tell those who are tormented and contorted by pain to stop assailing the gods with piteous pleas for a cure, and walk ten minutes each morning and evening on the bare earth, and drink in abundance fresh well water. Then they will become as they were and cease to trouble the gods.' It was, he said, a reference to the evil spirits that possess men and women. The Bible contains many mentions of evil spirits being cast forth from sufferers.

Of course, primitive people did not entirely believe that inimical supernatural beings had entered a person's body and given rise to madness, epilepsy or arthritis. They just offered that as the only explanation they could think of.

We found this of great interest and discussed it for some weeks until I remembered that my mother was unable to wear a lovely silver chain necklace that she once had given to her. After as little as half an hour it was tangled around her neck and needed rearranging.

Some statistics in China tend to show that more rich people than poor people suffer from epilepsy and various rhemuatic disorders. This is of interest when one realizes that rich Chinese people, child or adult, never under any circumstances leave their homes without wearing shoes and that their shoes are invariably felt-soled. Felt is one of the most effective non-conductors of electricity known.

Some time later, in Australia, we were introduced to a thirty-four-year-old man who had contracted rheumatoid arthritis and was by then virtually crippled. He had been a highly regarded competitive tennis player, and was the son of a director of a big manufacturing firm He had had every tretment that money could buy but he was getting worse, and his forthcoming marriage had been postponed.

We told him all about our theory of static electricity and he became enthusiastic and determined to try it. He walked, or rather hobbled, barefoot for fifteen minutes on the lawn at his home four times every day and even went so far as to have his shoes adapted, by having thin innersoles of silver made to fit into his shoes, with six thin silver pegs hammered into each sole so that they contacted the inner silver sole. His socks then had a piece cut out of each foot so that he was, literally, earthed.

It was just over a year before we heard of him again — we had by then completely forgotten him! He had got our address from a mutual friend and wrote to say that he was now married and was playing tennis again.

This may be considered a digression, but we have included it because we implicity believe that rheumatoid and osteoarthritis can be relieved. Observe we say **relieved** and not cured. The possibilities, of course, depend upon the stage reached in the disease before this treatment is attempted. The herbalist has no magic potions at his command. Nevertheless, he has available herbs therapeutic properties of which are proven, and these can inculcate considerable benefits for the sufferer.

We were requested years ago by many people living overseas to supply herbal medication that could help them with their arthritic problems. As we were unable to meet them we could not evaluate for ourselves their true condition, nor could we know what side-effects arising from their arthritis were troubling them. All we knew was that they were greatly concerned by the pain and crippling effects.

In ancient times in China, when an important man was ill, he might send a message to a famous doctor who enjoyed a high reputation for the treatment of the particular illness. To save time, if he considered the matter urgent, the doctor would pack every medicine that he thought could help in a parcel and send it off at once; and, because every town had its customs and municipal officers, he would plainly mark it 'Celestial Favour'. Nobody ever impeded this swift carriage of medicines. The doctors let it be known that any person who did would contract the illness of the patient if his death resulted.

We decided, therefore, to follow the same sensible practice and to send in one parcel everything that we confidently knew could help alleviate arthritis and allied conditions. We packed a selection of our most effective tablets and a special herbal compound made up to the following formula:

Avena Sat.	40%
Tarax Off.	15%
Ilex Para.	30%
Turnera Diff.	15%

That was ten years ago, and although we have always positively stated that we believed a **cure** for arthritis is impossible, and that the course can do no more than relieve pain and increase mobility, it has been an astounding success. We send it to all parts of the world and receive many requests for information.

Rheumatism

The name is used to identify many associated disorders, the primary cause of which is still unknown. One just cannot say 'I have rheumatism and it was caused by ....' The most that one can do is to state the symptoms accurately.

Nevertheless, it is one of the most widespread disorders of the world. Some estimates are that as many as 32 per cent of people over the age of forty are to some extent suffering from this disorder.

Rheumatism is painful, and can be incapacitating and crippling. The only thing that is definitely known about it is that there is no known certain cure. We believe that it is the resultant symptom of a long-endured primary malfunction. In simple words, we think something has disturbed the normal life processes of the individual and given rise to secondary manifestations and conditions that are known by the generic name of 'rheumatism'.

This, of course, is pure speculation, for we do not know (indeed, it is not our business to know, for herbalists are not doctors. They are concerned with herbs and the effects of herbs on the human body and not with the pathology of the individual). However, we do think that our years of experience and observation are of value in the treatment of rheumatism.

We claim nothing more than that certain herbs administered in specific doses can have some postive results in a high percentage of cases. This statement excludes any claim that we can **cure** rheumatism, or that we understand the nature of rheumatism. We cannot and we do not.

We believe that, frequently, conditions likely to give rise to rheumatoid conditions are exacerbated by neuroses which terminate in rheumatism. Just as the failure of an electrical transformer can plunge a city into darkness, so can nervous tension cause prolonged malfunction of the physiology of the body.

The quickest relief we can offer for all rheumatoid disorders is afford by this tablet made up as follows:

Guaiacum resin	60mg
Capsicin BPC 1923	15mg
Oil Celery	0.0005ml

and the aqueous extractive from

| Blue Flag | 135mg |
| Cascara | 90mg |

Sciatica

Sciatica is usually due to displacement of the cushioning cartilage between the vertebrae, which then presses upon the sciatic nerve endings. The location of the pain, which can be agonizing, is usually the buttocks, the backs of the thighs or the legs, and the most satisfactory therapy is rest.

The patient should rest and relax in a warm, draught-free place and eat very light but sustaining meals and of course drink plenty of simple fluids. If the pain is unusually severe. the patient's mattress should be supported by a board so that it will not yield too much to his weight.

It helps to massage the affected parts gently with a bland herbal balm and dry off with talcum powder. The balm we recommended is excellent but expensive to make. We also recommend that patients should take a herbal sciatica tablet:

Burdock		
Yarrow		
Bogbean	of each	30mg
Agrimony		
Raspberry Fol.		
Pot. Tart. acid		
Guaiacum resin	of each	15mg
Nutmeg		
Sulphur Sub		120mg

This formula is quick to act.

Varicose Ulcers and Varicose Eczema

We consider it significant that these are found most commonly on the lower leg, principally on the skin where there is least flesh. Its prevalence is confined to older persons, usually women who have borne several children. Rest is obviously the best therapy, and we advise all sufferers to rest as much as possible, and when resting to raise the leg as high as possible. We do not as a rule recommend wearing elastic stockings, as we consider that these can delay healing and cause ulcers to appear lower in the leg. The ulcer should be lightly bandaged and not in any way be constricted.

We use an ointment for the treatment of these complaints that is antiseptic and chemically hygiene. The formula is:

Calamine	12.50%
Strong Coal Tar soln.	2.50%
Zinc oxide	12.50%
Marshamallow root	0.50%
Comfrey root	0.50%
Slippery Elm bark	0.50%
Hydrous wool fat and white soft paraffin to	100.00%

We also recommend tablets made up as follows:

Motherwort	60mg
Hamamlidis	30mg
Chlorophyll 10%	15mg
Hydrastis	8mg
Rutin	8mg

and the aqueous extractive from

Uva Ursi	60mg

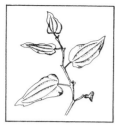

Part Two

Encyclopedia of Medicinal Herbs

Introduction

In collating this section we have endeavoured to be
practical. We have tried to include every herb of medicinal
value that may be procured through trade sources. At the
same time, since the book is intended to be a working tool
rather than a scholarly reference work, we decided that the
emphais should be on the **uses,** past and present, of these
herbs. The plants from which they come, therefore are not
always described in sufficient detail to enable an amateur to
gather them without recourse to a guidebook for
identification.**It must be stressed that anyone wishing to use
herbs gathered in the wild must be sure of their
identification.**

When a medicinal herb is identified by other than its
Latin name, it must always be suspect. The early settlers in
the colonies named new birds, flowers and plants after
similar ones in their home countries and much confusion
resulted. What is more, a lot of the confusion in common
names was, in fact, quite deliberate. Most of the
eighteenth-century herbalists were anxious to preserve the
secrets of their formulation and so named the principle
ingredients in such a manner that no other herbalist could
identify them. They also ground them into minute particles
so that they could not be recognized, and adulterated them
with some innocuous herbal matter with a strong odour, so
that any distinctive characteristics would be swamped.

'Strength Root', for example, was the asparagus root
(Asparagus officinalis). 'Egyptians leaves', much prescribed
by gypsies at fairgrounds, were the commonly known
coltsfoot leaves **(Tussilago farfara).** Perhaps the most
expensive herb ever sold in London was 'Moonleaves', which
was sold by a hairdresser in Cheapside for \$5 an ounce (that
would be about \$30 today). He seems to have implied that it
would safely and infallibly terminate pregnancies. After his
death 'Moonleaves' were discovered to be dried, ground
mistletoe leaves **(Viscim album).**

We are presently in the process of compiling a list of all local and common plant names now or formerly used throughout the world, along with their positive Latin equivalents. (This will not include Asian languages other than Hindi or Tamil for we are not able to cope with translations.) If any reader knows of any old local names for medicinal herbs and can positively state the modern common name for them, we would be very pleased to hear from him. Any such correspondence should be addressed to us at Cathay of Bournemouth Limited, 32 Cleveland Road, Bournemouth, UK. When writing, if possible enclose a few leaves from the plant.

Finally, one should remember that the rarity or **reported** virtues of many foreign herbs do not prove their efficacy. In fact, since the demand for any **proven** medicinal herb would most certainly quickly exhaust the supply, it is reasonable to assume that most of these reputed wonder herbs are of little importance and that their value is built upon 'travellers' tales'.

Abscess Root (Polemonium reptans)
Also known as Sweatroot
Found wild United States from New York to Wisconsin and Scandinavia.
Appearance Small semi-prostrate plant, 8-9in (20.5—23cm) high; feathery leves, blue flowers. The rhizomes alone are used.
Therapeutic or culinary uses Taken to promote perspiration and clear phlegm from the bronchial tubes. The herb is also strongly astringent.

Acacia Bark (Acacia arabica)
Also known as Wattlebark
Found wild North Africa
Appearance Small sturdy tree of which the bark is used. It is hard and gnarled, with black outer surface, red-liner inner surface.
Traditional and/or reputed uses Formerly used for its astringent properties but now little used in medicine. Of great repute in ancient times, it is frequently referred to in the Bible.

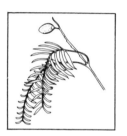

Acacia Gum (Acacia senegal)
Also known as Gum Arabic
Found wild North Africa
Appearance Round tears obtained from spring shrub. Descending cuts are made in the bark of the tree and the gum exudes and coagulates. When dry it is collected and exported to all parts of the world.
Therapeutic or culinary uses Acacia gum is an excellent and wholesome demulcent, and is often used to relieve catarrh and chest complaints.

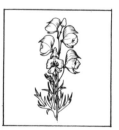

Aconite (Poisonous) (Aconitum napellus)
Also known as Monkshood, Wolfsbane, Blue Rocket
Found wild Southern Europe, Persia and as far east as China
Appearance A bold, dark, blue-violet-flowered herb of distinctive appearance. Up to 3ft (31 cm) high with dark green glossy leaves. Only the roots are used.
Therapeutic or culinary uses THIS PLANT IS POISONOUS, and no certain antidotes are known. It is used to allay nervous disorders and ease pain.
Authors' comments **Should not be used by Amateurs.**

Adder's Tongue (American) (Erythronium americanum)
Also known as Dog's Tooth Violet, Snake's tongue
Found wild North America from New Brunswick to Florida
Appearance Small bulbous plant with only two leaves; bright yellow, lily-like flowers, the leaf only is used.
Therapeutic or culinary uses Generally used as a poultice for ulcers and skin troubles.

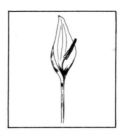

Adder's Tongue (English) (Ophioglossum vulgatum)
Also known as Christ's Spear
Found wild Throughout Great Britain in water meadows and swamps
Appearance Small single curling-leaved fern. The leaves only are used.
Therapeutic or culinary uses The fresh leaves make a most effective and comforting poultice for ulcers and tumours Also taken as an emollient for internal bleeding.

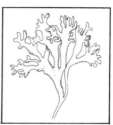

Agar-Agar (Gelidium amansii)
Also known as Japanese Isinglass
Found wild Japan
Appearance Agar-Agar is prepared from a compound of several different seaweeds collected from Japanese waters. It is imported in the form of thin strips about 12in (31cm) long.
Therapeutic or culinary uses Known to be excellent for the relief of stubborn constipation as it can absorb up to 160 times its own weight in water. however, it is principally used in scientific cultures and commerce.

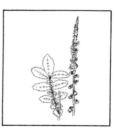

Agrimony (Agrimonia eupatoria)
Also known as Church Steeples, Sticklewort
Found wild Throughout northern Europe
Appearance A strong growing herb with greenish-grey leaves covered with soft hairs. Flowers are small and yellow and are displayed in long slender spikes. The leaves are used.
Therapeutic or culinary uses The dried leaves when infused make a mild and satisfying astringent useful for diarrhoea; also used as a tonic and diuretic.

Alder (American) (Prinos verticillatus)
Also known as Feverbush, Winterberry
Found wild North America from New Brunswick to Florida
Appearance A small tree, 6-10ft (2—3.5m) in height with white flowers. Bears red berries in profusion, similar to holly. The bark is used.
Therapeutic or culinary uses The bark when infused is a strong and reliable cathartic without any griping action.

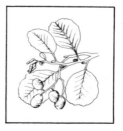

Alder (English) (Alnus glutinosa)
Found wild Throughout England, Europe and North Africa, usually in areas with a high water table
Appearance An attractive small tree of distinctive appearance. The small catkins after the seeds have ripened are called 'berries'. Both the bark and the leaves are used.
Therapeutic or culinary uses The bark is used as a cathartic and the leaves are used to treat inflammation.

Almonds (Prunus communis)
Also known as Sweet Almonds, Bitter Almonds, Turkey Almonds
Found wild Asia Minor and throughout the Middle East. It also grows freely in Britain.
Appearance A beautiful and familiar tree of medium size with alternate toothed leaves. The nuts are used.
Therapeutic or culinary uses Bitter almonds when distilled yield an essential oil containing about 5 per cent of prussic acid. Almonds are usually processed to extract almond oil for cosmetic purposes. Little is used for medicinal purposes, but almond flour is sometimes used as sustaining food for diabetics.

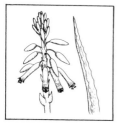

Aloes (Aloe vera)
Also known as Cape Aloes, Zanzibar Aloes, West Indian Aloes
Found wild Throughout southern Africa and West Indies.
Appearance A fleshy spiny or prickly succulent plant, of medium height; evergreen. The sap is used.
Therapeutic or culinary uses The sap when dried to powder makes a renowned purgative and expellent of intestinal worms. Also used to promote the menses.
Traditional and/or reputed uses A plant famous for its beneficial and curative properties from ancient times.

Alstonia Bark (Alstonia constricta)
Also known as Fever Bark, Australian Quinine
Found wild Australia
Appearance Thick chocolate-coloured spongy bark, stripped from a moderate-sized tree which grows in dry upland areas.
Therapeutic or culinary uses Commonly used in the Antipodes to prevent the recurrence of bouts of malaria. Also highly regarded as a specific for the quick relief of rheumatism in most of its forms.

Amaranth (Amaranthus hypochondriacus)
Also known as Love Lies Bleeding, Velvet Flower, Red Cockscomb
Found wild Europe ((but widely cultivated throughout the world)
Appearance A delicate plant with finely divided foliage and crimson flowers. Grows 4-5ft (1-2 metres) tall. The flowers are used.
Therapeutic or culinary uses Of great value for the safe treatment of diarrhoea and menorrhagia. Also used for sponging sores and ulcers.

Ammoniacum (Dorema ammoniacum)
Also known as Gum Ammoniacum
Found wild Turkey, Persia
Appearance Small rounded lumps, pale yellow in colour, browning with age. The gum resin is used.
Therapeutic or culinary uses Chiefly used for respiratory troubles. Excellent for the relief of catarrh, asthma or bronchitis.
Traditional and/or reputed uses Also highly regarded as an energy stimulant.

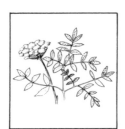

Angelica (Angelica archargelica)
Also known as Garden Angelica
Found wild Throughout Europe (also cultivated)
Appearance A stately garden plant with small, light green flowers. Grows up to 6ft (2 metres) in height. The roots, seeds and herb are all used.
Therapeutic or culinary uses Infusions are generally used to promote the flow of urine and expel wind. Also an excellent stimulant, and promotes perspiration. Chiefly used in decorative confectionery.
Authors' comments A delightful plant to grow in any garden.

Angostura (Galipea officinalis)
Also known as Angostura Bark, Cusparia Bark
Found wild South America
Appearance A diminutive hardy tree. Bark, stripped annually, has a musty tobacco-like odour.
Therapeutic or culinary uses A tonic. May also be used as a safe cathartic. However, it is almost always used to make an aromatic 'bitter' to heighten the flavour of gin.

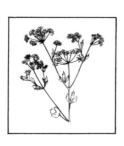

Aniseed (Pimpinella anisum)
Found wild European countries bordering the Mediterranean Sea and North Africa
Appearance An umbelliferous plant with much serrated leaves. Small, brownish-grey seeds have a strong pleasant odour, and a sweet spicy taste.
Therapeutic or culinary uses A pectoral. The distinctive flavour makes it a favourite ingredient for use in cough medicines and elixirs. It is most effective and quite safe for children.

Areca Nut (Areca catechu)
Also known as Botel Nut
Found wild India and Malaysia
Appearance Variety of palm tree. The nuts are large and similar to nutmeg.
Therapeutic or culinary uses A powerful astringent; also used to expel tapeworms.

Arenaria Rubra (Lepigonum rubrum)
Also known as Sandwort
Found wild Malta and Corsica
Appearance A small, low-growing plant with small pink
flowers. The leaves are infused.
Therapeutic or culinary uses Diuretic. Of great value for the
treatment of cystitis and stones.

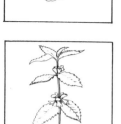

Arbutus, Trailing (Epigaea repens)
Also known as Mayflower, Ground Laurel
Found wild North America
Appearance Procumbent herb. Evergreen leaves, white
fragrant flowers. The leaves and stem are used.
Therapeutic or culinary uses A diuretic. Regarded as one of
the most effective palliatives for urinary disorders.
Authors' comments Especially recommended for the aged.

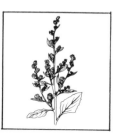

Archangel (Lamium album)
Also known as White Deadnettle
Found wild Throughout Great Britain
Appearance Similar to the common nettle but with a greyish
appearance, distinguished by its white flowers. The leaves
and stem are used.
Therapeutic or culinary uses A diuretic, for which purpose it
is excellent, and a most pleasant tonic.

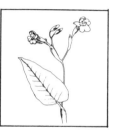

Arrach (Chenopodium olidum)
Also known as Goat's arrach, Stinking arrach
Found wild Throughout Europe
Appearance A small inconspicuous herb having an
unpleasant odour. The leaves and stems are used.
Therapeutic or culinary uses Principally used as an
emmenagogue to bring on menstruation. Also an effective
nervine
Authors' comments Justly regarded as one of the most
beneficial herbs.

Arrowroot (Maranta arundinacea)
Also known as Maranta St Vincent
Found wild West Indies and South America
Appearance A bold plant, up to 6ft (2 metres) in height. It
reproduces itself from spreading fleshy rhizomes, which are
powdered for use.
Therapeutic or culinary uses Famous for its pleasant
nutritional qualities. Also esteemed as a soothing
demulcent.
Authors' comments One of the most palatable foods for
invalids.

Asafoetida (Ferula foetida)
Also known as Devil's Dung
Found wild Persia and foothills of the Himalayas
Appearance Grows in bold clumps, 7ft (2¼ metres) high.
The gum resin is extracted from the fleshy roots. Odour
foetid, like garlic.
Therapeutic or culinary uses A stimulant and antispasmodic
of known virtue. Often used to relieve croup and colic. Also
used for sauces and flavourings.

Asarabacca (Asarum europaeum)
Also known as Hazelwort, Wild Nard
Found wild Brittany and northern Europe
Appearance A tall-growing perennial plant with
insignificant purple flowers. The root and leaves are used.
Therapeutic or culinary uses A strong emetic. A little sniffed
up the nostrils induces violent sneezing and a heavy flow of
mucus.
Authors' comments Not often used in medicine now.

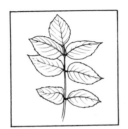

Ash (Fraxinus excelsior)
Also known as Common Ash, Weeping Ash
Found wild Throughout the Northern Hemisphere
Appearance A handsome, decorative tree of moderate size.
The bark and leaves are used.
Therapeutic or culinary uses Decoctions made from the
bark and leaves are a gentle laxative. Taken regularly, the
ash is said the prevent the recurrence of bouts of malaria. It
is also said to be excellent for the treatment of arthritic
conditions.

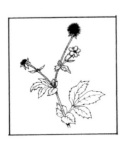

Avens (Geum urbanum)
Also known as Geum, Colewort
Found wild Throughout Europe
Apearance A low-growing herb with yellow flowers. The
seeds affix themselves to all who brush against them. The
roots and leaves are used.
Therapeutic or culinary uses Used to stay bleeding, it is a
strong astringent and a most reliable tonic, particularly for
women. It is also most useful for the treatment of
leucorrhea.

Azedaracha (Melia azedirachta)
Also known as Bead Tree, Pride of China
Found wild Afghanistan and northern India, and southern
United States
Appearance A large tree. Only the bark is used.
Therapeutic or culinary uses Its only medicinal use now is to
expel worms from children.

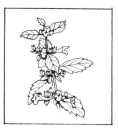

Balm (Melissa officinalis)
Also known as Lemon Balm, Sweet Balm
Found wild Throughout Europe
Appearance A plant, 2-3ft (½-1 metre) in height, with a lemon odour. The leaves are used.
Therapeutic or culinary uses Most effective for the relief of flatulence and indigestion and induces copious perspiration. Can also be made up into a most pleasant and cooling tea.

Balm of Gilead (Populus candicans)
Also known as—This can cause confusion as several other plants are known as Balm of Gilead.
Found wild United States. Arabia.
Appearance A strong, gnarled shrub with feathery foliage. The buds are used.
Therapeutic or culinary uses Highly regarded as a tonic. Also has diuretic properties. Made into pastilles or an ointment, it is most excellent for chest troubles and rheumatic ailments.
Authors' comments Balm of Gilead has been prized from the most ancient times. The true balm is derived from a small shrub.

Balmony (Chelone glabra)
Also known as Turtle Head, Snake Herb
Found wild Eastern United States and Canada
Appearance A low sturdy bush with crowded, oval dark leaves with spikes or white or pink flowers. The leaves are used.
Therapeutic or culinary uses Taken as an infusion, it is regarded as one of the best remedies for diseases of the liver. It is also antibilious, anthelmintic and a tonic.

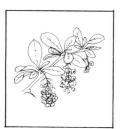

Barberry (Berberis vulgaris)
Also known as Barbery
Found wild Throughout Europe
Appearance A tall-growing straggling bush with very short thorns. Beautiful orange flowers in spring. The roots and berries are used.
Therapeutic or culinary uses Excellent for liver complaints and biliousness, and also a mild purgative.
Recommendations One of the safest of medicinal herbs.

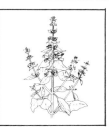

Basil (Ocimum basilicum)
Also known as Sweet Basil
Found wild Northern Europe
Appearance A small plant, with a multitude of white and pink flowers, whose leaves have a strong clover-like scent. The leaves are used.
Therapeutic or culinary uses Formerly used as a carminative but now almost only used for culinary purposes.

Bayberry (Myrica cerifera)
Also known as Waxberry, Candleberry, Wax Myrtle
Found wild Europe and North America
Appearance A medium-growing shrub with a profusion of
large white berries. The bark is used.
Therapeutic or culinary uses The bark yields one of the
strongest stimulants. It is warming, and justly regarded as
one of the most effective deobstruents and cleansers. It is
also comforting when used in poultices for applying to
ulcers.
Authors' comments One of the most useful herbs known to
science.

Bearsfoot, American (Polymnia uvedalia)
Also known as Yellow Leaf Cup
Found wild North America
Appearance A tall branching plant found in rich loamy soil.
The root is used.
Therapeutic or culinary uses Regarded as a valuable aid for
quick pain relief. It is also a gentle laxative, especially good
for the aged, and a stimulant.

Belladonna (Atropa belladonna)
Also known as Deadly Nightshade
Found wild Throughout Europe
Appearance A small bushy plant bearing shining black
fruits. The roots and leaves are used.
Therapeutic or culinary uses A narcotic, a mydriatic, and a
diuretic.
Authors' comment **This plant is poisonous, and very
dangerous!**

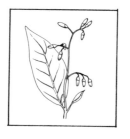

Benzoin (Styrax benzoin)
Also known as Gum Benzoin, Gum Benjamin
Found wild Far East
Appearance A sturdy tree of moderate size with
plum-coloured leaves. The gum is taken from wounds made
in the bark of the tree.
Therapeutic or culinary uses Infusions help to clear matter
from the bronchial tubes. It is one of the best expectorants,
and is an ingredient of Friars Balsam. It also has stimulant
properties.

Berberis (Berberis aristata)
Found wild India
Appearance Small shrub, grows freely in dry places. The
stem is used.
Therapeutic or culinary uses A valuable general tonic for
sufferers from malaria or fevers.

Beth Root (Trillium pendulum)
Also known as Woman's Root, Indian Shamrock
Found wild North America
Appearance A slender herb of low growth with abundant rhizomes emerging from the soil. The rhizomes alone are used.
Therapeutic or culinary uses Will allay excessive menstruation and it has been proved effective for menorrhagia. It is also a valuable astringent and tonic.

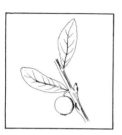

Bilberry (Vaccinium myrtillus)
Also known as Whortleberry, Hurtleberry
Found wild Great Britain
Appearance Grows in marshlands. A smallish plant with blue-black spherical berries. The berries are used.
Therapeutic or culinary uses A reliable diuretic. Also used for dysentry.
Traditional and/or reputed uses Formerly regarded as an excellent treatment for gravel.

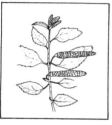

Birch (European) (Betula alba)
Also known as Birch
Found wild Europe
Appearance A strikingly handsome tree common on gravel soils. The distinctive black and white bark is used.
Therapeutic or culinary uses Birch tar oil, makes up into a soothing ointment for skin disorders and eruptions. The bark, when taken as an infusion, is good for kidney stones.

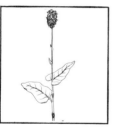

Bistort (Polygonum bistorta)
Also known as Adderwort, Dragonworth
Found wild Northern countries of Great Britain and Europe
Appearance Low-growing herb chiefly found in ditches and damp places. The root is used.
Therapeutic or culinary uses Regarded as a sure cure for incontinence. It is often used as a gargle for sore throats.
Traditional and/or reputed uses A very strong astringent and highly styptic.

Bitter Apple (Citrullus colocynthis)
Also known as Colocynth, Bitter Cucumber
Found wild Middle East
Appearance Annual plant resembling a watermelon. The fruit pulp is used.
Therapeutic or culinary uses A very violent purgative and so strong that it is mostly used only in combination with other herbs.

Bitter Root (Apocynum androsaemifolium)
Also known as Dogsbane, Fly Trap
Found wild North America
Appearance A woody herb with acuminate leaves. The roots are used.
Therapeutic or culinary uses Famous as a safe cathartic and heart tonic; it is also a powerful emetic and diuretic.
Traditional and/or reputed uses Supposed in olden times to ensure the recovery of those bitten by mad dogs.
Authors' comments Not to be confused with Gentian, which is also known as bitter root.

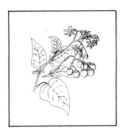

Bittersweet (Poisonous) (Solanum dulcamara)
Also known as Woody Nightshade
Found wild Throughout Britain
Appearance A weak-growing nondescript climber. The twigs and the bark off the roots are used.
Therapeutic or culinary uses Used as an infusion, it is excellent for relieving rheumatic or arthritic pains. Also highly regarded as a diuretic and has strong narcotic properties.
Authors' comments **This plant is poisonous.**

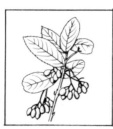

Black Haw (Viburnum prunifolium)
Also known as American Sloe
Found wild United States
Appearance Shrub with gamopetalous flowers and acuminate leaves. The root bark is used.
Therapeutic or culinary uses This is an excellent tonic for women, particularly those who fear they may suffer a miscarriage. It is an effective nervine and often taken as a sedative.

Black Root (Leptandra virginica)
Also known as Physic Root, Culver's Root
Found wild United States
Appearance A low-growing herb of which the rhizomes only are used.
Therapeutic or culinary uses Its principle use is in blood-purifying mixtures. Also used as a cathartic, a diaphoretic (its action is always mild and pleasant) and a liver stimulant.

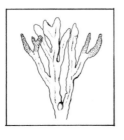

Bladderwrack (Fucus vesiculosus)
Also known as Seawrack or Kelpware
Found wild Around the coasts of Britain
Appearance A very large trailing seaweed, very dark green in colour, and with the fronds made buoyant by paired oval bladders. All of it is used.
Therapeutic or culinary uses Chiefly used as the principle agent in 'cures' for obesity. It is also said to clean out the kidneys and to tone up the system. It is one of the most prolific sources of natural iodine and trace elements.

Blood Root (Sanguinaria canadensis)
Also known as Red Root
Found wild Canada and northern United States
Appearance A significant member of the poppy family. the rhizomes alone are used.
Therapeutic or culinary uses Has strong, quick-acting stimulant properties and is one of the best remedies for the relief of chronic bronchitis and pneumonia. Heavy doses act speedily to quell whooping cough and croup.
Traditional and/or reputed uses Used as a tincture, it clears up ringworm.

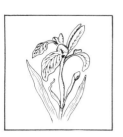

Blue Flag (Iris versicolor)
Also known as Flag Lily, Water Flag
Where found Extensively planted in gardens throughout Britain.
Appearance A beautiful plant with arching, strap-like leaves and blue, white, yellow or multi-coloured flowers. The rhizomes alone are used.
Therapeutic or culinary uses The principle agent in most blood-purifying compounds, it acts as an alterative, diuretic and cathartic.

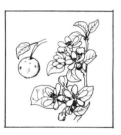

Blue Mallow (Malva sylvestris)
Also known as The Mallow
Found wild Throughout Europe
Appearance A boldly growing herb with alternate leaves, and bright blue, many-petalled flowers. The flowers and leaves are used.
Therapeutic or culinary uses Regarded as one of the best demulcents, it is used in a very high proportion of all cough cures. Especially recommended for children.

Boldo (Penmus bodus)
Also known as Boldu
Found wild Chile
Appearance Medium-sized shrub with dark oval leaves and a strong lemon smell. The leaves only are used.
Therapeutic or culinary uses Mostly used as a liver stimulant, it also has antiseptic properties and is of great value to sufferers from catarrh of the bladder.

Boneset (Eupatorium perfoliatum)
Also known as Feverwort, Thoroughwort
Found wild Northern Hemisphere
Appearance A small, low-growing herb 3-4ft (1-1¼ metres) in height. All of the plant is used.
Therapeutic or culinary uses regarded as one of the surest remedies for fevers and influenza. It is also a tonic and a laxative, and can be taken as an expectorant.

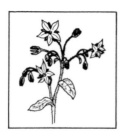

Borage (Borago officinalis)
Also known as Burrage
Found wild Throughout Europe
Appearance Bold, erect herb of strong growth. Small blue flowers. The leaves are used.
Therapeutic or culinary uses Usually used as a flavouring agent in cordials and cooling drinks. It is also a diuretic and demulcent.
Authors' comments this is a plant that will give pleasure in any garden.

Boxwood (American) (Cornus florida)
Also known as Dogwood, Cornel
Found wild United States
Appearance A small tree with very rough bark and a profusion of pink flowers in spring. The bark and root bark are used.
Therapeutic or culinary uses A powerful tonic and stimulant and said to be one of the most reliable remedies for migraine and headaches.

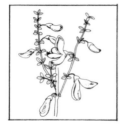

Broom (Cytisus scoparius)
Also known as Irish Broom, Sarothamnus Genista
Found wild Throughout Europe
Appearance A small, graceful arching shrub. Profuse floral display. The tips only are used.
Therapeutic or culinary uses A herb most highly regarded from ancient times for its excellent diuretic and cathartic qualities. Frequently taken with excellent results for the relief or liver troubles and fluid retention.

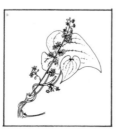

Bryony, Black (Tamus communis)
Found wild Great Britain
Appearance Any untidy climbing plant with alternate leaves. The roots are used.
Therapeutic or culinary used It used to be freely used, when rubbed on flesh, to relieve rheumatic and arthritic pains and gout. It is also an effective diuretic. Externally a popular remedy for black eyes and bruises. It is little used now.

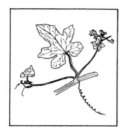

Bryony, White (Bryonia dioica)
Also known as Lady's Seal, Mandragora
Found wild Throughout Europe
Appearance A large-leaved climbing plant of the cucumber family. The roots only are used and they are very large, white and fleshy.
Therapeutic or culinary uses Posseses a very strong hydrogogue and cathartic action, it is also useful for chest disorders. Should be taken only when prescribed by experts, as the effects can be dangerous.
Authors' comments This herb is in no way related to Black Bryony.

Buchu (Barosma betulina)
Also known as Bucco
Found wild Western coast of South Africa
Appearance A small, procumbent herb growing in dry places. The leaves are used.
Therapeutic or culinary uses One of the most beneficial of all medicinal herbs. Excellent and quickly effective for urinary troubles, gravel and catarrh of the bladder. It is also a diaphoretic and stimulant.

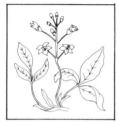

Buckbean (Menyanthes trifoliata)
Also known as Bogbean, Water Trefoil
Found wild Throughout Europe
Appearance Small herb, grows in damp and marshy places. All of it is used.
Therapeutic or culinary uses A celebrated tonic, very popular in medieval times for the treatment of rheumatism and gout. It is also effective for skin diseases.

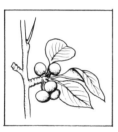

Buckthorn (Rhamnas cathartica)
Found wild Europe and North Africa
Appearance A small spreading tree. The berries only are used.
Therapeutic or culinary uses The juice is a strong laxative; formerly popular, but now used only in animal husbandry.

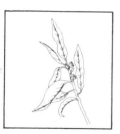

Buckthorn Alder (Rhamnus frangula)
Found wild Europe and United States
Appearance A small tree of irregular growth. The dried young bark only is used.
Therapeutic or culinary uses A tonic and cathartic liable to cause griping pains if taken in too concentrated a dose.

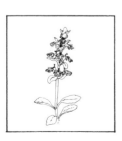

Bugle (Ajuga reptans)
Also known as Sicklewort
Found wild European woodlands
Appearance A diminutive herb with distinctive square stems. Blue flowers. The leaves are used.
Therapeutic or culinary uses An astringent, but little used now.

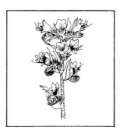

Bugloss (Echium vulgare)
Also known as Viper's Bugloss
Found wild Europe
Appearance A sturdy herb with blue flowers. The leaves are used.
Therapeutic or culinary uses An expectorant and demulcent. Excellent for evacuating the bowels without griping effect. It is also taken to clear phlegm from the bronchial tubes.

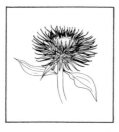

Burdock (Arctium lappa)
Also known as Cockle Buttons
Found wild Throughout Europe
Appearance A small, strong-growing herb of distinctive appearance. The roots, seeds and leaves are used.
Therapeutic or culinary uses A powerful diaphoretic, it is also an effective diuretic and possesses sedative properties. Justly regarded as one of the best blood purifiers.

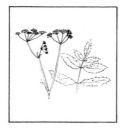

Burnet, Greater (Sanguisorba officinalis)
Also known as Garden Burnet
Found wild Great Britain
Appearance An erect purplish flowered herb. The leaves are used.
Therapeutic or culinary uses Formerly highly regarded as a tonic, it has now lapsed from favour. Can also be used as an astringent, for which pupose it is most effective.
Traditional and/or reputed uses Useful in diarrhoea and dysentry.

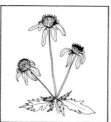

Burr Marigold (Bidens tripartita)
Also known as Water Agrimony
Found wild Europe
Appearance Procumbent plant that forms large colonies. All of the plant is used.
Therapeutic or culinary uses Normally used to relieve disorders of the respiratory system and to stem bleeding and haemorrhages. It is also a most valuable diaphoretic, with astringent properties.

Bush Tea (Cyclopia genistoides)
Also known as Rooibosch (Afrikaans, meaning Red Bush)
Found wild South Africa
Appearance A small erect bush of striking appearance. The leaves are used.
Therapeutic or culinary uses Often dried and drunk as tea in South Africa. Also of great value to sufferers from kidney and liver disorders.

Calamint (Calaminta officinalis)
Also known as Common Calamint, Mountain Mint
Found wild Throughout Europe
Appearance A small, low-growing herb with purple flowers.
The leaves are used.
Therapeutic or culinary uses An expectorant and
diaphoretic usually made up into syrup or linctus. Not
commonly used now.

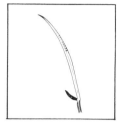

Calamus (Acorus calamus)
Also known as Sweet Flag
Found wild Throughout Europe, near water
Appearance A hardy aquatic plant. The rhizomes alone are
used.
Therapeutic or culinary use Excellent for flatulence and all
forms of stomach disorders.

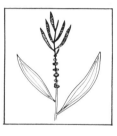

Cajuput (Melaleuca leucadendron)
Also known as White Tea Tree
Found wild East Indies
Appearance A big bold tree. The oil only is used.
Therapeutic or culinary uses Usually made up into lotions
and ointments. It is excellent for all forms of rheumatism
and bruises and gives comfort when rubbed on to the gums
for sufferers from toothache. A few drops taken on sugar
quickly ends hiccoughs.

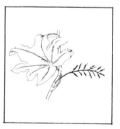

Calumba (Jateorhiza palmata)
Also known as Colombo
Found wild East Africa
Appearance One of the palm family, of undistinguished
appearance. The root only is used.
Therapeutic or culinary uses Chiefly taken to relieve
stomach disorders, for it is a valuable tonic and stomachic.
Also a powerful febrifuge.

Canadian Hemp (Apocynum cannabinum)
Also known as Black Indian Hemp
Found wild United States and Canada
Appearance A small laurel. The roots and rhizomes are
used.
Therapeutic or culinary uses Little used in Europe, it is
favoured in North America for the treatment of
amenorrhoea and leucorrhoea. It is also of value for its
diaphoretic and emetic properties.

Canella (Canella alba)
Also known as Wild Cinnamon
Found wild West Indies
Appearance A slender branching tree with light grey bark, which alone is used.
Therapeutic or culinary use A most effective stimulant and tonic for the aged. It promotes digestion and elimination and prevents flatulence.

Caraway (Carum carvi)
Also known as Caraway Seed
Found wild, Europe and North Africa
Appearance A hollow-stemmed herb usually grown in plantations. The seeds are used.
Therapeutic or culinary use A favourite flavouring. Expecially recommended for children.

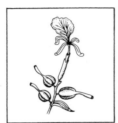

Cardamom (Elettaria cardamomum)
Also known as Malabar Cardamom
Found wild Ceylon
Appearance A boldly growing plant of exotic appearance. The seeds are used.
Therapeutic or culinary uses Its warming, aromatic, stomachic action is most beneficial for sufferers from flatulence and indigestion. It is also used to give 'note' to fine curries.

Caroba (Jacaranda procera)
Also known as Carob Tree
Found wild South Africa and South America
Appearance A handsome tree with lanceolate leaves. The leaves are used.
Therapeutic or culinary uses Chiefly used by the natives, who prize it highly as a diaphoretic and diuretic. It is also a safe sedative.

Cascara Sagrada (Rhamnus purshiana)
Also known as Cascara
Found wild United States and Canada
Appearance A low-growing small tree. The bark only is used.
Therapeutic or culinary uses Regarded as one of the safest and most purely effective tonic laxatives.
Authors' comments The demand exceeds the supply!

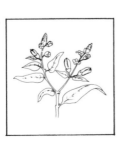

Cascarilla (Croton eleuteria)
Also known as Sweet Wood Bark
Found wild West Indies-Bahamas only
Appearance A diminutive tree. The bark is used.
Therapeutic or culinary uses A tonic and a stimulant, it has a safe and gentle action.

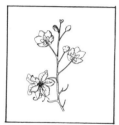

Cassia (Cinnamomum cassia)
Also known as Cassia Bark, Chinese Cinnamon
Found wild China
Appearance A strong-growing member of the laurel family.
The bark and buds are used.
Therapeutic or culinary use Much used in China and the
Far East as a tonic, stomachic and carminative, where it is
highly regarded. It as freely exported in pre-Christian times
and is several times mentioned in the Bible.

Cassia Pods (Cassia fistula)
Found wild Egypt and East Indies
Appearance A medium-sized tree with yellow scented
flowers. The pulp of the fruit is used.
Therapeutic or culinary uses A gentle, fruit-flavoured
laxative, usually put up with other laxatives as a compound.

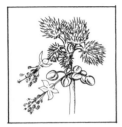

Castor Oil Plant (Poisonous Seeds) (Ricinus communis)
Also known as Palma Christi
Found wild Throughout the tropics.
Appearance A big shrub. The oil is used.
Therapeutic or culinary uses Regarded as the best of all
purgatives and especially favoured for children and the
aged. It is also used externally for itch and ringworm.
Authors' comments **The Seed is very poisonous.**

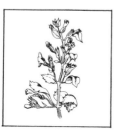

Catnip (Nepeta cataria)
Also known as Catmint
Found wild Great Britain
Appearance A procumbent grey plant usually grown as an
edging in gardens. The leaves are used.
Therapeutic or culinary uses Has distinct carminative,
diaphoretic and tonic properties. It is also made up into an
ointment for the relief of piles.

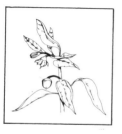

Cayenne (Capsicum minimum)
Also known as Chillies, Red Pepper, Bird Pepper
Found wild West Africa and tropical America
Appearance A small erect herb with brilliant dark green
foliage. The fruit only is used.
Therapeutic or culinary uses One of the best and most
positive stimulants known in herbal science. Also a
carminative and rubefacient of great value, and a valued
condiment.

Cayenne, Hungarian (Capsicum tetragonum)
Also known as Paprika
Found wild Hungary (also cultivated on a grand scale)
Appearance A strong-growing herb with large resplendent green fruits. The fruits are used.
Therapeutic or culinary uses One of the richest known sources of vitamin C, it is gaining in popularity in Britain where it is used in salads. Also excellent when boiled as a vegetable.
Traditional and/or reputed use Said to promotote longevity.

Cedron (Simaba cedron)
Found wild Central America
Appearance A small tree. The seeds only are used.
Therapeutic or culinary uses A bitter tonic and a febrifuge celebrated for its effeciency. Also regarded as a valuable draught for malaria.

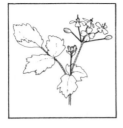

Celandine (Cheidonium majus)
Also known as Greater Celandine
Found wild Throughout Europe
Appearance A member of the poppy family. The leaves are used.
Therapeutic or culinary uses When taken as an infusion is most effective for clearing eczema and other scrofulous troubles. It is also a diuretic and a strong purgative.

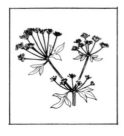

Celery (Apium graveolens)
Found wild Europe
Appearance This is the familiar vegetable. The seeds are used.
Therapeutic or culinary uses Always regarded as one of the most effective aphrodisiacs. It is also a tonic, diuretic and carminative and a most beneficial aid for the relief of rheumatoid troubles.
Authors' comments The seed must be collected before the plant has been frosted.

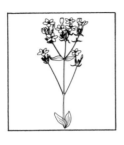

Centaury (Erythraea centaurium)
Also known as Feverwort
Found wild Europe and North Africa
Appearance A small, pink-flowered herb. The leaves are used.
Therapeutic or culinary uses A stomachic and aromatic tonic. Good for most stomach upsets and jaundice. A very bitter flavour.

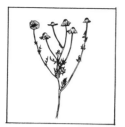

Chamomile (Anthemis nobilis)
Also known as Belgian Chamomile
Found wild Belgium and France (also widely cultivated)
Appearance A herb with double flowers. The flower is used.
Therapeutic or culinary uses One of the best remedies for women who suffer from nervous upsets, and regarded as one of the most reliable tonics. Also used as a stomachic and antispasmodic.

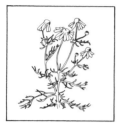

Chamomile (German) (Matricaria chamomilla)
Also known as Wild German Chamomile
Found wild Europe
Appearance A herb with small cushion-like flowers, produced in great profusion. The flowers are used.
Therapeutic or culinary uses Considered to be a most excellent nerve sedative, it is classified as a carminative, a sedative and a tonic.
Authors' comments Can also be used as a tisane.

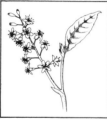
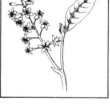

Cherry Laurel (Prunum laurocerasus)
Found wild Russia, Asia Minor
Appearance One of the larger members of the laurel family. The leaves only are used.
Therapeutic or culinary uses a reliable sedative and frequently the principal agent in cough medicine.

Chestnut (Castanea sativa)
Also known as Sweet Chestnut
Found wild Europe and America
Appearance A large tree of magnificent appearance. The leaves only are used.
Therapeutic or culinary uses A tonic and an astringent. When used to control paroxysmal coughing and whooping cough, its efficacy is remarkable and it is most soothing.

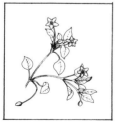

Chickweed (Stellaria media)
Also known as Starweed
Found wild Throughout Great Britain
Appearance A small prolific weed. The leaves alone are used.
Therapeutic or culinary uses A demulcent of proven value, and also used to allay feverish conditions.

Chiretta (Swertia chirata)
Also known as Indian Gentian
Found wild India
Appearance A small wiry herb growing freely in arid places. All of the plant is used.
Therapeutic or culinary uses An extremely bitter tonic which quickly restores a flagging appetite.

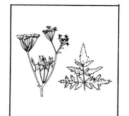

Cicely, Sweet (Myrrhis odorata)
Also known as Sweet Chervil
Found wild Throughout Great Britain
Appearance A very pretty, erect growing herb. The root and the leaves are used.
Therapeutic or culinary uses A herb with many uses. It is a carminative and an expectorant, and a fine tonic for young females. It is also used as a remedy for coughs and is regarded as excellent for those who suffer from anaemia.

Cineraria Maritima (Senecio maritimus)
Also known as Dusty Miller
Found wild West Indies (now cultivated in English gardens)
Appearance A small plant with finely divided silver leaves. The juice is used.
Therapeutic or culinary uses Its only medicinal use is for the treatments of cararacts of the eyes.

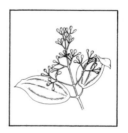

Cinnamon (Cinnamomum zeylanicum)
Found wild Ceylon
Appearance Another of the laurel family. An evergreen of noble appearance. The bark is used, rolled and dried in cylindrical quills.
Therapeutic or culinary uses As a carminative and stimulant it is indeed excellent, and it quickly ends vomiting. Also used as an aromatic and astringent and for culinary purposes as a flavouring and spice.
Traditional and/or reputed uses Highly regarded and exported from ancient times, it is referred to in the Bible.

Clary (Salvia sclarea)
Also known as Cleareye
Found wild Throughout Great Britain
Appearance A bold blue- or white-flowered herb that grows freely as a weed wherever it can get a start. The leaves are used.
Therapeutic or culinary uses Its most frequent use is to cleanse and refresh the eyes. It is an antispasmodic and is also used to relieve stomach and kidney disorders.

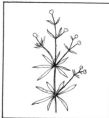

Clivers (Galium aparine)
Also known as Goosegrass
Found wild Throughout Great Britain
Appearance A rampant weed with lanceolate bristly leaves that is most difficult to eradicate from gardens. The leaves are used.
Therapeutic or culinary uses An aperient and diuretic of proven efficiency, it is also excellent for the dispersal of bladder stones.

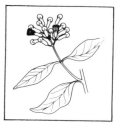

Cloves (Eugenia caryophyllus)
Found wild Zanibar, Madagascar and the East Indies
Appearance A beautiful evergreen tree of majestic stature. The unopened flower ends are used, by having the oil extracted from them.
Therapeutic or culinary uses A stimulant and carminative, usually compounded with other remedies. The oil is used in cosmetics and the untreated buds as a spice.

Clubmoss (Lycopodium clavatum)
Also known as Lycopodium
Found wild Northern Hemisphere
Appearance A low-spreading, greyish green, insignificant plant usually found near water. The plant and spores are used.
Therapeutic or culinary uses This plant offers great relief for cystitis and kidney diseases, and allied urinary disorders. It is also a reliable sedative and is excellent for the treatment of dyspepsia and stomach disorders.

Cohosh, Black (Cimicifuga racemosa)
Also known as Bugbane, Squawroot
Found wild United States and Canada
Appearance A procumbent spreading herb, very bitter and with a disagreeable odour. The rhizomes are used.
Therapeutic or culinary uses A powerful emmenagogue and diuretic. Usually prescribed for obstructed menses. It is also excellent for the treatment of whooping cough and fevers.

Cohosh, Blue (Caulophyllum thalictroides)
Also known as Blueberry Root
Found wild United States and Canada
Appearance A gnarled and crowded shrub. The rhizomes alone are used.
Therapeutic or culinary uses Used generally as a diuretic and emmenagogue, and as a vermifuge to expel worms. It is most highly regarded for its qualities in dealing with women's complaints. It also offers quick relief from pain to rheumatic sufferers.

Colchicum (dangerous) (Colchicum autumnale)
Also known as Meadow Saffron
Found wild Europe and North Africa.
Appearance Somewhat similar to a tulip, but growing from a corm, which alone is used.
Therapeutic or culinary uses Mostly used for the relief of rheumatic and gouty disorders. It is quick to act and most comforting.
Authors' comments **Should be taken in minute quantities, and then only if prescribed by a Herbalist!**

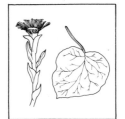

Coltsfoot (Tussilago farfara)
Also known as Coughwort
Found wild Throughout Europe, usually near water.
Appearance A small bright green herb. The flowers appear before the leaves. Both flowers and leaves are used.
Therapeutic or culinary uses Used in cough mixtures and is regarded as one of the most effective herbs for this purpose known to science. The Romans stationed in Britain exported honey-flavoured cough medicines back to Rome. Coltsfoot is also used in herbal tabaccos to relieve chest troubles.

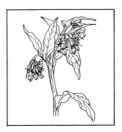

Comfrey (Symphytum officinale)
Also known as Knitbone, Slippery Root
Found wild Throughout Europe, usually near water.
Appearance A bushy plant with hairy green leaves. The root and the young leaves are used.
Therapeutic or culinary uses Best known for its great value in the treatment of pulmonary ills. It is also a valuable demulcent and astringent. It is used in poultices for the healing of ulcers and reduction of inflammations.

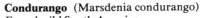

Condurango (Marsdenia condurango)
Found wild South America
Appearance A nondescript climbing vine indigenous to heavily forested areas. The bark alone is used.
Therapeutic or culinary uses An alterative and stomachic. Recent experimentation reveals that it is one of the best known drugs for duodenal ulcers.

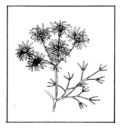

Coriander (Coriandrum sativum)
Found wild Southern Europe and the Near East
Appearance A diminutive herb. The fruit is used.
Therapeutic or culinary uses A valuable carminative taken to soothe and ease the bowels. Also acts as a stimulant to restore appetite and vigour. It is also a favourite flavouring.

Corn Ergot (Poisonous) (Ustilago maydis)
Also known as Cornsmut
Found wild South Africa and America
Appearance A fungus living on maize. The finely divided, dark coloured powder is used.
Therapeutic or culinary uses Highly regarded as an emmenagogue and parturient, it is also frequently used for menstrual troubles.
Authors' comments **Corn Ergot is poisonous. Great care should be exercised in its usage.**

Corn Silk (Zea mays)
Found wild South Africa and America
Appearance The stigmas from the small female flowers of maize are used.
Therapeutic or culinary uses Principally used as a diuretic and regarded as one of the most effective. Also efficacious for pulmonary troubles.

Cotton Root (Gossypium herbaceum)
Found wild Mediterranean islands and United States
Appearance The bark is used medicinally and is sold in thin strips rolled into twists.
Therapeutic or culinary uses Of great value in the treatment of women's disorders. It contracts the uterus and promotes the menstrual flow. Also, it aids women whose sexual drive is lessened.

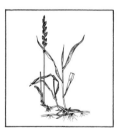

Coughgrass (Agropyron repens)
Also known as Twitchgrass
Found wild In most parts of the world (difficult to eradicate from gardens and cultivated places)
Appearance A strong growing grass with white fleshy roots. The rhizomes are used.
Therapeutic or culinary uses Most effective for the treatment of cystitis and nephritis and bladder troubles. Also excellent for the treatment of rheumatoid ills. It is a diuretic and aperient.
Authors' comments One of the safest and most effective of herbal remedies.

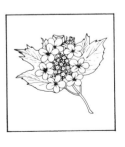

Cramp Bark (Viburnum opulus)
Also known as Snowball Tree, Guelder Rose
Found wild Europe and America
Appearance A strong-growing bush with white ball-shaped flowers. The bark is used.
Therapeutic or culinary uses Cramp Bark is an excellent nervine of particular value for the treatment of spasms and convulsions. It is also one of the best antispasmodics. Regarded as a particularly safe medication for children's use.

Cranesbill (American) (Geranium maculatum)
Also known as Wild Geranium, Storksbill
Found wild United States
Appearance Small shrubby herb with blue flowers. The root
is used.
Therapeutic or culinary uses Famous for its quick styptic
properties, it is also a tonic and astringent. Useful for piles
and internal ulcers.

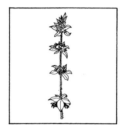

Crosswort (Galium cruciata)
Also known as Yellow Bedstraw
Found wild Throughout the British Isles
Appearance A small yellow-flowering herb. The stem and
leaves are used.
Therapeutic or culinary uses Once widely used for treating
wounds and staunching the flow of blood.

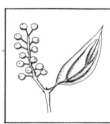

Cubeb (Piper cubeba)
Also known as Tailed Pepper
Found wild Far East
Appearance A small, very quick-growing vine. The
unripened fruit is used.
Therapeutic or culinary uses An aromatic and expectorant,
it is a valuable remedy for catarrh and lung disorders.

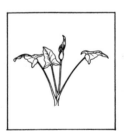

Cuckoopint (Poisonous) (Arum masculatum)
Also known as Lords and Ladies, Wake-Robin
Found wild Europe
Appearance A distinctive shield-like single leaf encloses the
bright red berries. The root is used.
Therapeutic or culinary uses Noted as a diaphoretic and
expectorant. And old remedy but in little use today.
Authors' comments **Should not be taken unless prescribed
by a qualified Herbalist, for it can be poisonous!**

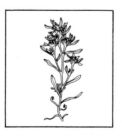

Cudweed (Gnaphalium uliginosum)
Also known as Cottonweed
Found wild Europe
Appearance A small weed of prolific growth, preferring dry
soil. The whole plant is used.
Therapeutic or culinary uses An astringent, usually taken
with excellent results, to cure quinsy. Can also be used as a
gargle.

Cumin (Cuminum cyminum)
Found wild North Africa and the Nile.
Appearance An erect and handsome herb with feathery foliage. The fruit is used.
Therapeutic or culinary uses A carminative. A favourite veterinary medicine for horses that are 'blown' through eating fresh spring grass.

Damiana (Turnera diffusa)
Found wild Southern United States and Mexico
Appearance The leaves only are used.
Therapeutic or culinary uses Famous for its aphrodisiac qualities (it is generally regarded as one of the best and most effective in the world). It is also a wonderful tonic, and can be given with safety to the senile and those suffering from exhaustion and debility, particularly to people recovering from influenza.

Dandelion (Taraxacum officinale)
Found wild In most temperate climates
Appearance A common herb with a long root, toothed leaves and bright yellow flowers.
Therapeutic or culinary uses A tonic and a diuretic, justly regarded as one of the most reliable remedies for liver and kidney ills. The roots are frequently used as a substitute for coffee — many think it preferable, as it contains no caffeine.

Deer's tongue (Liatris odoratissima)
Also known as American Wild Vanilla
Found wild United States
Appearance A strong-growing climbing plant with obovate-lanceolate leaves. The leaves are used.
Therapeutic, or culinary use A powerful stimulant, highly regarded by the North American Indians as an aphrodisiac, and said to induce erotic dreams. Also a most effective diuretic.

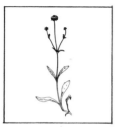

Devil's Bit (Scabiosa succisa)
Found wild British Isles
Appearance An insignificant purplish plant. The whole plant is used.
Therapeutic or culinary uses Excellent as an infusion for coughs and chest inflammation. Also a reliable demulcent and a diaphoretic.

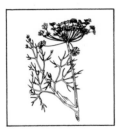

Dill (Anethum graveolens)
Also known as Dill seed
Found wild Europe
Appearance An elegant erect herb with distinctive flowers stems. The dried fruit is used.
Therapeutic or culinary uses One of the earliest medicinal herbs known in Europe. It is very effective for conditions of flatulence and dyspepsia and its carminative and stomachic qualities are well attested.
Authors' comments One of the best remedies of its kind for young children.

Dodder (Cuscuta epithymum)
Found wild Throughout the world
Appearance A climbing parasite of the convolvulus family. The stem and leaves are used.
Therapeutic or culinary uses A mild laxative and a well regarded hepatic, it is of value for the treatment of bladder and liver troubles.

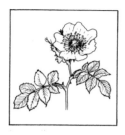

Dog Rose (Rosa canina)
Also known as Wild Briar
Found wild Europe and Middle East
Appearance The wild rose. The hips are used.
Therapeutic or culinary uses The hips yield ascorbic acid (vitamin C) and are of the greatest value when given to young children.
Traditional and/or reputed uses One of the best tonics for old dogs.

Dragon's Blood (Daemonorops propinquus)
Found wild Malaya
Appearance A dwarf member of the palm family. The resin is used.
Therapeutic or culinary uses A stringent, and regarded as effective for the treatment of dysentery. Much used in magical rituals.

Echinacea (Echinacea angustifolia)
Also known as Coneflower
Found wild United States
Appearance A herb of medium height. The rhizomes are used.
Therapeutic or culinary uses An antiseptic and alterative. Regarded by the North American Indians as one of the very best blood-purifying herbs. It is also used for typhoid.

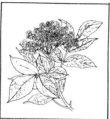

Elder (Sambucus nigra)
Also known as Black Elder
Found wild Europe
Appearance A tall, straggling shrub with profuse crops of black berries. All the herb is used.
Therapeutic or culinary uses A great favourite of the early Saxon for colds and influenza. It is an alterative and diuretic. Elderberry wine is a safe soporific and induces healthy sleep.

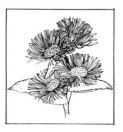

Elecampane (Inula helenium)
Found wild Europe and Asia
Appearance A bold perennial plant with long divided roots. The root alone is used.
Therapeutic or culinary uses A powerful expectorant and a valuable ingredient in cough mixtures. It also has effective diaphoretic and diuretic properties. It makes up into a fine complexion wash.

Embelia (Embelia ribes)
Found wild India
Appearance Similar to a stunted redcurrant bush. The fruits are used.
Therapeutic or culinary uses It has taenicide properties and is used by Indians to expel tapeworms.

Ephedra (Ephedra sinica)
Also known as Ma Huang
Found wild The cold areas of China and Mongolia
Appearance A tall-growing plant with graceful arching fronds. The stems are used.
Therapeutic or culinary uses A most valued herb for the relief of asthma. A nervine and tonic.

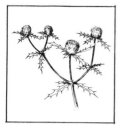

Eryngo (Eryngium campestre)
Also known as Sea Holly
Found wild Europe
Appearance A small procumbent herb. The root is used.
Therapeutic or culinary uses A diaphoretic and expectorant. It also promotes the flow or urine and eases bladder irritation and diseases.

Euphorbia (Euphorbia hirta)
Found wild Tropical Asia
Appearance A small shrub with bristly stems. The stem and leaves are used.
Therapeutic or culinary uses This herb is regarded as offering the quickest relief from asthma. It is much used in the Antipodes where it is considered indispensable.

Euphorbium (Euphorbia resinifera)
Found wild North Africa
Appearance A shrub of dense growth with fleshy stems. The dried sap is used.
Therapeutic or culinary uses A violent purgative.

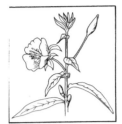

Evening Primrose (Oenothera biennis)
Also known as Tree Primrose
Where found A European garden plant
Appearance A small herb with a delightful early display of yellow flowers. The leaves and bark are used.
Therapeutic or culinary uses A sedative of proven value and also an astringent. Is reliably used to relieve female menstrual disorders.

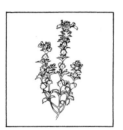

Eyebright (Euphrasia officinalis)
Found wild Europe
Appearance A diminutive insignificant herb with tiny whitish flowers. The stem and leaves are used.
Therapeutic or culinary uses Mostly used as a lotion for eye troubles, for which it is most comforting and efficient. Lotions for this purpose are exported to all parts of the world.

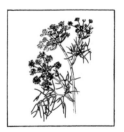

Fennel (Foeniculum vulgare)
Found wild Mediterranean countries and warmer parts of Britain
Appearance A tall annual herb with dainty foliage. The seeds are used.
Therapeutic or culinary uses Generally used to flavour liquorice powder. A gentle and reliable carminative and stomachic, it also has stimulant properties. Excellent for flavouring fish dishes.

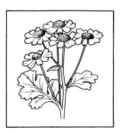

Feverfew (Chrysanthemum parthenium)
Also known as Featherfew
Found wild Throughout Europe
Appearance A small grey herb with hairy stems. The stems and leaves are used.
Therapeutic or culinary uses This herb is an easy aperient without any griping action, and it has always been favoured by women to bring on the menses.

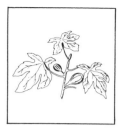

Figs (Ficus carica)
Found wild Throughout the Mediterranean countries and Near East
Appearance A medium-sized tree of rampant growth. The fruit is used.
Therapeutic or culinary uses Since ancient times infusions of figs have been taken as an aperient. They are also emollient and demulcent and are useful when used in a hot poultice for ulcers.

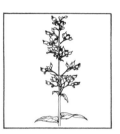

Figwort (Scrophularia nodosa)
Also known as Throatwort
Found wild Throughout Europe
Appearance A medium-sized herb. The stem and leaves are used.
Therapeutic or culinary uses Used as a poultice to cleanse and heal skin eruptions, abscesses and ulcers. It is an anodyne and eases pain wherever it is applied.

Five-Leaf-Grass (Potentilla reptans)
Also known as Fivefinger
Found wild Throughout Great Britain
Appearance A small procumbent herb. The root and leaves are used.
Therapeutic or culinary uses Makes up into a useful astringent lotion. Taken as an infusion, it reduces fevers. It also acts to correct diarrhoea.

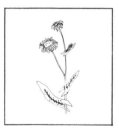

Fleabane (Erigeron canadense)
Also known as Coltstail
Found wild Europe and North America
Appearance A small, low-growing herb with white flowers. The leaves and seeds are used.
Therapeutic or culinary uses A tonic and diuretic, usually taken for gravel and kidney troubles.

Fluellin (Linaria elatine)
Found wild Throughout Europe in dry regions
Appearance A small spreading recumbent plant with tiny yellow flowers. The leaves are used.
Therapeutic or culinary uses Considered an infallible remedy for menstrual flooding.

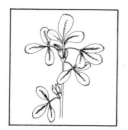

Foenugreek (Trigonella foenum-graecum)
Also known as Fenugreek
Found wild North Africa
Appearance A tall graceful plant 2-3ft (½-1 metre) in height. The seeds are used.
Therapeutic or culinary uses An emollient used in poultices. It is also taken as an infusion to soothe stomach inflammation. A valuable flavouring agent for culinary uses.

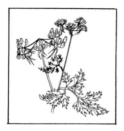

Fool's Parsley (Poisonous) (Aethusa cynapium)
Also known as Dog Parsley
Found wild Throughout Europe
Appearance A small herb distinguished by triple slender leaves below flower clusters. The leaves are used.
Therapeutic or culinary uses This herb is not related to the true parsley and it **Can be both toxic and dangerous to use.** It is a sedative and stomachic but should **be taken only when correctly prescribed!**

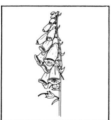
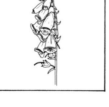

Foxglove (Poisonous) (Digitalis purpurea)
Also known as Purple Foxglove
Appearance A tall annual plant with purplish flowers. The leaves are used.
Therapeutic or culinary uses A valuable heart tonic, sedative and diuretic.
Authors' comments **This plant is poisonous and must not be taken unless prescribed!**

Fringetree (Chionanthus virginica)
Found wild Southern United States
Appearance A small tree with insignificant white flowers. The bark of the roots is used.
Therapeutic or culinary uses Excellent for the treatment of liver disorders, gallstones and female ills.

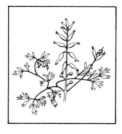

Fumitory (Fumaria officinalis)
Found wild Throughout Europe
Appearance A small low-growing herb. The stem and leaves are used.
Therapeutic or culinary uses A gentle aperient and an effective diuretic. Can also be used as an infusion to bathe skin eruptions.

Galangal (Alpinia officinarum)
Also known as East India Root
Found wild Southern China
Appearance Of similar appearance to a garden iris. The rhizomes are used.
Therapeutic or culinary uses One of the best of all herbs for the treatment of dyspepsia and persistent flatulence. It is also an effective stimulant. Also used as an unusual spice for flavouring dishes.

Galbanum (Ferula galbaniflua)
Also known as Gum Galbanum
Found wild Near East
Appearance A boldly growing shrub. The gum exudes from the stems and it is the gum resin that is used.
Therapeutic or culinary uses A stimulant, taken to relieve rheumatism and nervous paroxysms.

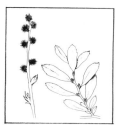

Gale Sweet (Myrica gale)
Also known as Bog Myrtle
Found wild Mediterranean countries
Appearance A low-growing herb, all of which is used.
Therapeutic or culinary uses An aromatic and astringent, it is also a most valuable hair tonic.

Galls (Quercus infectoria)
Also known as Oak Galls
Found wild Near East
Appearance A growth similar to a nutmeg, caused by an insect laying eggs within the bark of the tree. The gall is used.
Therapeutic or culinaary use An astringent, usually taken for the relief of dysentery and diarrhoea.
Traditional and/or reputed uses Has been used since ancient times for the preparation of leather — the galls contain a high percentage of tannic acid.

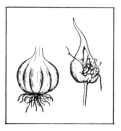

Garlic (Allium sativum)
Where found Universally cultivated
Appearance Similar to the shallot. The bulb is used.
Therapeutic or culinary use A most effective expectorant and diaphoretic. It is claimed that it also has an antiseptic effect upon the bowels. Garlic oil is much used in veterinary preparations.

Gelsemium (Gelsemium sempervirens)
Found wild Southern United States
Appearance A strong-growing climbing plant with delightfully scented yellow flowers. The root is used.
Therapeutic or culinary uses A strong and successful sedative and a valuable diaphoretic and antispasmodic. It is also used to allay toothache and neuralgia, and for women's disorders.
Authors' comments Most excellent for persons who are senile.

Gentian (Gentiana lutea)
Found wild Snow lines of Europe
Appearance A small rock plant with flowers of the most intense blue. The root is used.
Therapeutic or culinary uses Justly regarded as one of the best tonics known to medical science.

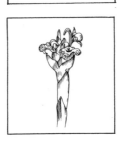

Gentian (English) (Gentiana campestris)
Also known as Field Gentian
Found wild Throughout Great Britain
Appearance Small herb with purple flowers. The root and leaves are used.
Therapeutic or culinary uses Similar to the true gentian, but very much less effective.

Ginger (Zingiber officinale)
Found wild West Indies and China
Appearance Height about 3ft (1 metre) with glossy aromatic leaves. Its fleshy roots are dried and peeled. The rhizomes only are used.
Therapeutic or culinary uses Justly famed for its stimulative and carminative properties; can also be used as an expectorant. It aids digestion and promotes a feeling of warmth and wellbeing. Ginger also forms the basis of many sauces and flavourings and is much used in confectionery.

Ginger, Wild (Asarum canadense)
Also known as Canadian Snakeroot
Found wild North America
Appearance A small herb that forms dense drifts on gravelly soil. The rhizomes are long and slender and they alone are used.
Therapeutic or culinary uses Wild ginger is in no way related to the true ginger: it is a member of the Aristolochiacea family. It is similar in effect to real ginger, but is a far quicker and more effective expectorant.

Ginseng (Panax quinquefolium)
Also known as Chinese Panacea, Panax, The Gift of the Gods
Found wild China and Mongolia
Appearance An erect growing herb with vivid fleshy leaves. The roots alone are used.
Therapeutic or culinary uses This is the oldest known medicine substance. It is recorded prior to 2000 BC. It has **properties as an effective aphrodisiac and is quite without** irritative after-effects. It is also a most effective tonic for the aged and senile and for sufferers from digestive troubles.
Authors' comments The genuine wild-grown roots are probably the most expensive herbs in the world.

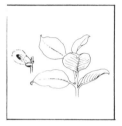

Goat's Rue (Galega officinalis)
Also known as Galega
Found wild Throughout Europe
Appearance About 12in (30cm) high, a member of the pea family. The stem and leaves are used.
Therapeutic or culinary uses One of the quickest and most effective vermifuges.

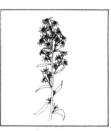

Goldenrod (Solidago virgaurea)
Found wild Throughout Great Britain (also widely cultivated)
Appearance A pretty garden plant with tall heads of golden bloom. The stem and leaves are used.
Therapeutic or culinary uses Chiefly taken for the relief of stomach ills. It is very efficient for flatulence and aids digestion. It has a general stimulant action.

Golden Seal (Hydrastis canadensis)
Also known as Yellow Root
Where found Cultivated in North America
Appearance A tall-growing herb with a most disagreeable and persistent odour. The rhizomes are used.
Therapeutic or culinary uses A herb of the very greatest value for the treatment of gastric disorders, it has a soothing laxative action. It is also a tonic and a detergent.

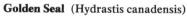

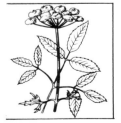

Goutwort (Aegopodium podagraria)
Also known as Goutweed
Found wild Throughout Europe
Appearance A small spreading herb. It is a nuisance in gardens and very difficult to eradicate. The leaves are used.
Therapeutic or culinary uses A sedative of peculiar virtues. When taken as an infusion it relieves sciatica and gout quickly. It is also a diuretic and of value when used as a poultice.

Gravel Root (Eupatorium purpureum)
Found wild United States
Appearance A low-growing herb of the dandelion family.
The rhizomes are used.
Therapeutic or culinary uses In America it is regarded as the
best treatment for stones in the bladder and kidney and
urinary troubles. It is safe and pleasant to use.

Grindelia (Grindelia camporum)
Found wild United States and South America
Appearance A low-growing sturdy herb with yellow flowers.
The stem and leaves are used.
Therapeutic or culinary uses This is a herb of proven
medicinal value. It is much used as a specific for relieving
asthma and bronchial troubles, and also given to children
for whooping cough. It is also a reliable diuretic.

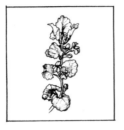

Ground Ivy (Glechoma hederacea)
Found wild Throughout Europe
Appearance One of the smaller ivys with very dark green
leaves. The stem and leaves are used.
Therapeutic or culinary uses Formerly much taken for
kidney troubles and for its tonic qualities. Also applied as a
compress for boils, abscesses and ulcers.

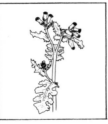

Groundsel (Senecio vulgaris)
Found wild Throughout the Northern Hemisphere
Appearance A semi-trailing small herb which grows
anywhere. The leaves and stem are used.
Therapeutic or culinary uses Taken as an infusion it
promotes profuse perspiration. It can also act as an emetic.

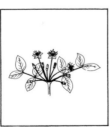

Guaiacum (Guaiacum officinale)
Also known as The famous Lignum Vitae
Found wild West Indies and South America
Appearance A strong tree producing the heaviest and
strongest wood in the world. Shavings and the gum are
used.
Therapeutic or culinary uses Considered to be one of the
most effective cures for rheumatism known. Its properties
are diaphoretic and alterative.

Guarana (Paulinia cupana)
Also known as Brazilian Cocoa
Found wild Brazil
Appearance A tall arching shrub. The seeds are roasted, pulped and used as a beverage.
Therapeutic or culinary uses A powerful stimulant, relieving headaches and migraines very quickly. It is also used by women to bring on the menses and is said to be effective for the treatment of arthritis.
Recommendations This herb contains a high percentage of caffeine.

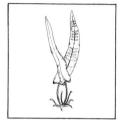

Hartstongue (Scolopendrium vulgare)
Found wild Europe
Appearance This is one of the more graceful ferns. The stem and leaves are used.
Therapeutic or culinary uses A diuretic and strong laxative. Taken as a weak infusion, it is quick to relieve congestion and lung inflammation. It also allays hiccoughs.

Hawthorn (Crataegus oxycantha)
Also known as May Tree
Found wild Throughout Britain
Appearance A common small tree. The berries are used.
Therapeutic or culinary uses The hawthorn is justly claimed to be one of the most effective aids for heart conditions. It is a tonic of the very greatest value for all sufferers from heart ailments.

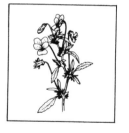

Heartsease (Viola tricolor)
Also known as The Wild Pansy
Found wild British Isles
Appearance Similar to the garden pansy with small purple and white flowers. The stems and leaves are used.
Therapeutic or culinary uses Used for the relief of catarrh and chest congestion and regarded as one of the best children's remedies. Also much used in blood-purifying mixtures.

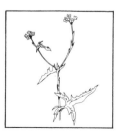

Hedge Mustard (Sisymbrium officinale)
Found wild Throughout the Northern Hemisphere
Appearance A straggling plant with light green leaves and small yellow flowers. The leaves are used.
Therapeutic or culinary uses Formerly much used to relieve colds and influenza. It is said to be excellent for the relief of laryngitis.

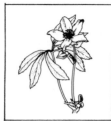

Hellebore Black (Helleborus niger)
Also known as Christmas Rose
Where found Throughout Europe (cultivated widely)
Appearance This is the delightful garden plant that flowers in January each year. The rhizomes only are used.
Therapeutic or culinary uses Its principal use is as an emmenagogue and of great value to women who suffer from period disorders. It is, as well, a most effective stimulant for those suffering from nervous depressions.

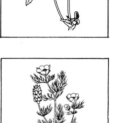

Hellebore, False (Adonis vernalis)
Also known as Peasant's Eye
Found wild Europe and Asia
Appearance A small plant with a large yellow flower. All of the herb is used.
Therapeutic or culinary uses Regarded as effective for the relief of most cardiac troubles. It is also a tonic and a diuretic.
Authors' comments **Should be taken only when prescribed by a qualified Herbalist.**

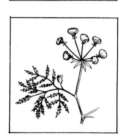

Hemlock (Poisonous) (Conicum maculatum)
Also known as Poison Hemlock
Found wild Europe
Appearance A tall herb with long strip-like leaves. The leaves and fruits are used.
Therapeutic or culinary uses Hemlock is a quick and powerful anodyne and also a strong sedative. Its medicinal uses are for the relief of nervous spasms and mental upsets. It is a notorious poison and was used in biblical times to put prisoners out of their miseries.
Authors' comments **Take only when prescribed.**

Henbane (Poisonous) (Hyoscyamus niger)
Also known as Hogbean
Found wild Europe
Appearance A strong-growing perennial plant with a profusion of yellow flowers. The leaves and small flowers are used.
Therapeutic or culinary uses Its effects are very similar to hemlock, but it is a stronger narcotic and can give rise to insensibility more quickly.
Authors' comments **This plant is poisonous and should be taken only when prescribed.**

Henna (Lawsonia alba)
Found wild Middle East and India
Appearance A strong plant of erect growth with distinctive leaves. The leaves only are used.
Therapeutic or culinary uses This is the plant famous from the earliest times for its qualities as a dye. It is also much used as an astringent.

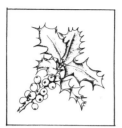

Holly (Ilex aquifolium)
Fould wild Throughout Europe
Appearance A small tree with glossy, shiny-eyed leaves, bearing a profusion of red or yellow berries in winter. The berries and flowers are used.
Therapeutic or culinary uses Used mostly to relieve chest troubles and laryngitis.
Traditional and/or reputed uses Reputed to be effective for the treatment of rheumatoid disorders.

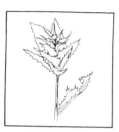

Holy Thistle (Carbenia benedicta)
Found wild Southern Europe
Appearance A typical thistle. The stem and leaves are used.
Therapeutic or culinary uses A safe emmenagogue and diaphoretic, useful in cough medicines. It was much used by Roman women for menstrual troubles.

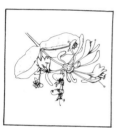

Honeysuckle (Lonicera caprifolium)
Found wild Throughout Europe
Appearance A strong climbing plant with deliciously scented flowers. The flowers and leaves are used.
Therapeutic or culinary uses A safe and excellent expectorant which quickly cleans the lungs. It is also a gentle laxative with a beneficial liver action.

Hops (Humulus lupulus)
Found wild Europe (and now cultivated in most temperate parts of the world)
Appearance A climbing vine. The flowers are used.
Therapeutic or culinary uses One of the most useful of plants. It quickly eases pain by virtue of its properties as an anodyne. It is a tonic, is good for most stomach disorders, and promotes sleep. It is also used to preserve beer and add to its flavour.

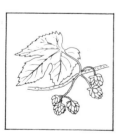

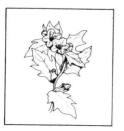

Horehound (Marrubium vulgare)
Found wild Europe and Britain
Appearance A strong erect herb with square stems. The stems and leaves are used.
Therapeutic or culinary uses One of the most effective expectorants known, it is used in most cough mixtures to clear phlegm. It is also a fine tonic.

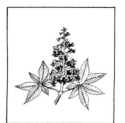

Horse Chestnut (Dangerous) (Aesculus hippocastanum)
Where found Cultivated in every temperate climate
Appearance A magnificent deciduous tree of noble proportions
Therapeutic or culinary uses A tonic, but now little used for this purpose. It is also a narcotic and a febrifuge, and is claimed to be good for the treatment of rheumatoid ills.
Authors' comments **Some caution must be exercised in its use.**

Horsemint (Monarda punctata)
Found wild United States
Appearance A small herb, one of the mint family. The leaves are used.
Therapeutic or culinary uses Is much taken for the relief of stomach disorders. Women use it as an emmenagogue.

Horsenettle (Solanum carolinense)
Found wild A common member of the nettle family. The roots and berries are used.
Therapeutic or culinary uses A sedative and antispasmodic. Of very great value for the treatment of juvenile convulsions and hysterical conditions in women arising from menstrual disorders.

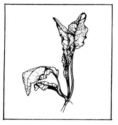

Horseradish (Cochlearia armoracia)
Found wild Europe
Appearance A herb growing up to 3ft (1 metre) tall with a pungent odour. The roots are used.
Therapeutic or culinary uses Warms and relieves flatulence and indigestions. It also promotes perspiration and is an excellent diuretic.

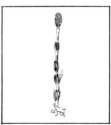

Horsetail (Equisetum arvense)
Also known as Scouring Rushes
Found wild Great Britain
Appearance A tall bold herb with a cane-like appearance. The leaves are used.
Therapeutic or culinary uses This herb is a powerful astringent and also possesses diuretic properties. It is excellent for kidney troubles. It has a strong abrasive action and is much used for polishing and scouring.

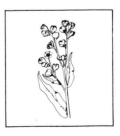

Houndstongue (Cynoglossum officinale)
Found wild Great Britain
Appearance A medium-sized herb with long, strap-like leaves. The stem and leaves are used.
Therapeutic or culinary uses An anodyne that quickly relieves pain, and is also a demulcent with soothing properties for the cure of coughs and colds. Can also be used to reduce piles.

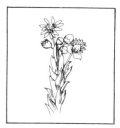

Houseleek (Sempervivum tectorum)
Found wild Throughout Great Britain
Appearance A small procumbent plant. The young leaves are used.
Therapeutic or culinary uses It has cooling properties when used as a poultice and it is an astringent. Is commonly used to soften and alleviate corns and hard skin.

Hydrangea (Hydrangea aborescens)
Also know as The Seven Barks
Found wild United States (this is not the cultivated garden hydrangea.
Appearance Similar to the common hydrangea. The roots are used.
Therapeutic or culinary uses A strong purgative, but in lesser doses it is a most valuable nephritic and removes gravel and stones from the bladder.

Hydrocotyle (Hydrocotyle asiatica)
Also known as Indian Pennywort
Found wild Tropical India and Africa
Appearance A small plant similar to angelica. The leaves are used.
Therapeutic or culinary uses Claimed in India as one of the most quickly effective aphrodisiacs for the middle-aged, it is wholesome and safe to use. It is also beneficial for the treatment of urinary disorders.
Authors' comments The demand now exceeds the supply.

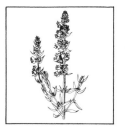

Hyssop (Hyssopus officinalis)
Found wild Throughout Great Britain
Appearance A small, prolific herb common in fields and meadows. The leaves only are used.
Therapeutic or culinary uses Compounded with other herbs, this makes a most excellent cure for colds and bronchial congestion.

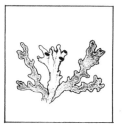

Iceland Moss (Cetraria islandica)
Found wild Throughout the Northern Hemisphere
Appearance This is **not** a moss, but a procumbent grey lichen. All of it is used.
Therapeutic or culinary uses Regarded as a certain cure for chronic catarrh and bronchitis. It is a nutritive and is helpful when taken with a diet prescribed for sufferers from digestive complaints.

Indian Hemp (Dangerous) (Cannabis sativa)
Also known as Dagga, **Ganjah**
Found wild Middle East
Appearance A tall-growing herb with serrated leaves.
Therapeutic or culinary uses Remarkably efficient for dispelling nervous depression and nervous spasms.
Authors' comments Illegal to use in Great Britain.

Indian Physic (Gillenia trifoliata)
Found wild United States
Appearance A member of the rose family, it grows into a straggling bush about 7ft (2.33 metres) high. The bark of the roots is used.
Therapeutic or culinary uses This is the poor man's Ipecacuanha, and was the principal constituent of 'cure-all' nostrums sold by travelling medicine salesmen in America. It is an expectorant, a cathartic and an emetic and is good for the treatment of constipation, coughs, dropsy and dysentery. It was even better for the salesmen, who sold so much that it became known as the 'Dime a bottle' plant.

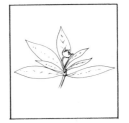

Ipecacuanha (Cephaelis ipecacuanha)
Found wild South America
Appearance A beautiful, elegant and exotic plant. The root alone is used.
Therapeutic or culinary uses One of the most beneficial of all plants. A most effective expectorant and widely used for chest and bronchial troubles. It is also a very quick emetic.
Authors' comments Ipecacuanha is used in literally thousands of proprietary and ethical medicines.

Irish Moss (Chondrus crispus)
Also known as Carragheen Moss
Found wild Below tide level on European and North American coasts
Appearance A small procumbent seaweed with fan-shaped fronds. All of it is used.
Therapeutic or culinary uses Used mainly in cough medicines for its excellent demulcent and pectoral qualities. Is also a counter-irritant to combat bladder and kidney troubles. It is nutritious and can be used as a food.

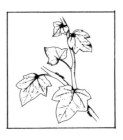

Ivy (Hedera helix)
Also known as Common Ivy
Found wild Europe
Appearance The self-clinging, evergreen climbing plant. The berries and leaves are used.
Therapeutic or culinary uses A strong stimulant but also a purgative. Was once used as a specific in poultices for ulcers and abscesses. It was believed to be a cure for the plague.

Jaborandi (Pilocarpus microphyllus)
Found wild Brazil
Appearance A small herb. The leaves are used.
Therapeutic or culinary uses A very strong diaphoretic and expectorant, it is most beneficial for the relief of asthma, and is often used to help sufferers from diabetes. It is also known to be one of the most effective agents for restoring hair losses.

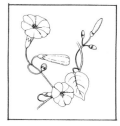

Jalap (Ipomaea purga)
Found wild South America
Appearance A robust climbing plant. The root is used.
Therapeutic or culinary uses Jalop is one of the most effective purgatives known to science and is universally prescribed.

Jamaican Dogwood (Dangerous) (Piscidia erythrina)
Found wild West Indies and Atlantic coast of South America
Appearance A small tree. The bark is used.
Therapeutic or culinary uses It is an anodyne and much used to relieve pain. It is a quick sedative and excellent for relieving nervous tension.
Authors' comments **This should be taken only when prescribed, — it can be dangerous!**

Jambul (Eugenia jambolana)
Also known as Java Plum
Found wild East India
Appearance A large spreading tree. The seeds are used.
Therapeutic or culinary uses One of the most effective drugs for diabetics. It quickly reduces urinal sugar content.

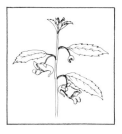

Jewel Weed (Impatiens aurea)
Found wild East Indies
Appearance A small dry herb. The leaves are used.
Therapeutic or culinary uses An aperient and a diuretic. It is of value for the relief of piles, and is also used to remove warts and corns.

John's Bread (Ceratonia siliqua)
Also known as Locust Beans
Found wild The Middle East
Appearance A strong and sturdy tree bearing in profusion the long brown pods which alone are used.
Therapeutic or culinary uses Used since biblical times to relieve prostate troubles. Also known for nutritional value.
Traditional and/or reputed uses In the last century all opera singers took this daily to improve their voices.

Jujube (Zizyphus vulgaris)
Found wild North Africa and the Middle East
Appearance A shrub that commonly grows in dry places.
The berries are used.
Therapeutic or culinary uses Famous for many thousands of
years as a specific for the cure of colds and bronchial
troubles. It was made up into lozenges and widely exported.
Some lozenges are still called 'jujubes'

Juniper (Juniperus communis)
Found wild Northern Hemisphere
Apearance A conifer tree. The berries are used.
Therapeutic or culinary uses Juniper is an excellent
stimulant and is of particular value to women and those
suffering from kidney disorders. Juniper berries are also
used to flavour gin.

Kamala (Mallotus philippinensis)
Found wild India and Arabia
Appearance A low-growing tree. The outer covering of the
fruits is dried and powdered for use.
Therapeutic or culinary uses Regarded as one of the most
effective agents for the expulsion of tapeworms.

Kava Kava (Dangerous) (Piper methysticum)
Found wild Fiji
Appearance A lofty shrub. The root is used.
Therapeutic or culinar uses A strong stimulant with
valuable tonic properties. Also has diuretic qualities and is
used to relieve conditions of incontinence.
Traditional and/or reputed uses It can be fermented and
used as an intoxicant liquor. **Taken too freely it produces
Hallucinations.**

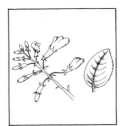

Kino (Pterocarpus marsupium)
Also known as Gum Kino
Found wild India and Ceylon
Appearance A very large tree of noble and magnificent
appearance. The sap is used.
Therapeutic or culinary uses An effective astringent.

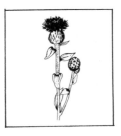

Knapweed (Centaurea nigra)
Also known as Ironweed
Found wild Great Britain
Appearance A small herb. The leaves are used.
Therapeutic or culinary uses It is a strong tonic and a
diaphoretic and diuretic, but is infrequently used now.

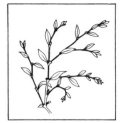

Knotgrass (Russian) (Polygonum erectum)
Found wild Russia
Appearance A small herb. The leaves are used.
Therapeutic or culinary uses An astringent. Also excellent for relieving children's diarrhoea.

Kola (Cola vera)
Also known as Kola Nut, Cola Nut
Found wild West Africa
Appearance A large tree of outstanding elegance. The seed is used.
Therapeutic or culinary uses Celebrated for its aphrodisiac powers, it is also a nerve stimulant and heart tonic. It promotes strength and endurance and is justly regarded as one of the very best stimulants. Now used to make up a popular soft drink.

Kumarhou (Pomaderris elliptica)
Found wild The North Island of New Zealand
Appearance A very pretty shrub. The herb is used.
Therapeutic or culinary uses Regarded by the Maoris as a universal panacea, it is said to be very good for the treatment of rheumatism and pulmonary disorders. Also used to purify the blood.

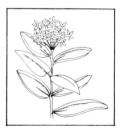

Labrador Tea (Ledum latifolium)
Found wild North America
Appearance A small bitter herb, all of which is used.
Therapeutic or culinary uses A reliable diuretic with pectoral and expectorant properties. Much used by the Red Indians.

Lachnanthes (Lachnanthes tinctoria)
Also known as Spirit Plant
Found wild West Indies
Appearance A small herb with protruberant snake-like rhizomes. The rhizoms and leaves are used.
Therapeutic or culinary uses A hypnotic and a stimulant of peculiar value to the aged. It is used in voodoo and magical formulae.

Lady's Bedstraw (Galium verum)
Found wild Great Britain
Appearance A small herb with pretty yellow flowers. The leaves are used.
Therapeutic or culinary uses A diuretic and excellent for the treatment of gravel and kidney stones.

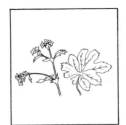

Lady's Mantle (Alchemilla vulgaris)
Found wild Great Britain
Appearance A low growing herb with tiny green flowers.
The leaves are used.
Therapeutic or culinary uses Of great value to women who
use it to allay menstrual flooding. It is also a styptic and
astringent.

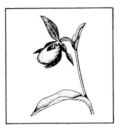

Lady's slipper (Cypripedium pubescens)
Also known as Nerveroot
Found wild Europe and United States
Appearance This is the delicate wild orchid. The rhizomes
are used.
Therapeutic or culinary uses A most effective nervine and
widely used to allay disorders of nervous origin. It also
induces healthy natural sleep.

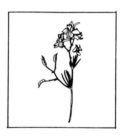

Larkspur (Delphinium consolida)
Also known as Common Larkspur
Found wild Throughout Europe
Appearance The common blue-flowering plant. The seeds
are used
Therapeutic or culinary uses A strong parasiticide. In
medieval times was regarded as the best delousing agent.
Tincture of Larkspur was an army issue to Wellington's
troops at Waterloo.

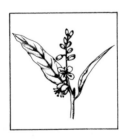

Laurel (Laurus nobilis)
Also known as Bay Tree
Found wild Europe
Appearance An evergreen tree with lanceolate leaves which
grows up to 25ft (8 metres) high. The leaves and fruit are
used.
Therapeutic or culinary uses The laurel wreathes given to
Victors at the Olympic Games were made of this tree. It is a
stomachic and the oils are used in liniments for the relief of
rheumatism.

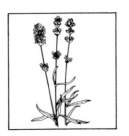

Lavender (Lavandula officinalis)
Found wild The Mediterranean area and Great Britain (also
cultivated)
Appearance A favourite garden plant which grows to 3ft (1
metre) in height. It is distinguished by its grey needle-like
leaves. The flowers and oil are used.
Therapeutic or culinary uses It has some stimulant
properties and is an effective carminative. However,
lavender is chiefly used in the manufacture of cosmetics.

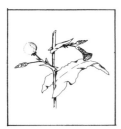

Lettuce, Wild (Lactuca virosa)
Found wild The warm parts of Europe
Appearance A small plant of bushy appearance. The dried juice is used.
Therapeutic or culinary uses An anodyne and sedative with hypnotic characteristics. It is also used to ease coughs of nervous origin.

Life Root (Senecio aureus)
Found wild Europe and North America
Appearance An erect herb with yellow flowers. The rhizomes and the herbs are used.
Therapeutic or culinary uses A most valuable herb indeed. It is an emmenagogue and is considered the best for bringing on the menses. It is also a pectoral with soothing beneficial properties, and a tonic of recognized value.

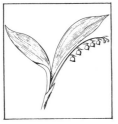

Lily Of The Valley (Convallaria majalis)
Where found Throughout Great Britain
Appearance The garden plant. All parts are used.
Therapeutic or culinary uses Highly recommended as a cardiac tonic with no after-effects. Strong doses act as a purgative.

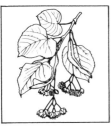

Lime Flowers (Tilia europoea)
Also known as Linden Flowers
Found wild Throughout Europe
Appearance A graceful tree. The flowers are used.
Therapeutic or culinary uses A strong but quite safe nervine for relief of headaches and hysteria. Also a stimulant and tonic.
Traditional and/or reputed used The Vikings spread the flowers on the floor of bridal bed chambers to ensure that the children should be tall and beautiful.

Linseed (Linum usitatissimum)
Also known as Flax Seed
Found wild Thoughout the world
Appearance An erect plant with strong fleshy leaves. The seeds are used.
Therapeutic or culinary uses Because of its valuable pectoral, demulcent and emollient qualities it is commonly used in cough medicines and poultices.

Lippa (Lippia dulcis)
Found wild Mexico
Appearance A spreading prostrate herb. The leaves are used.
Therapeutic or culinary uses A demulcent and expectorant of extraordinary efficiency. It is regarded as one of the most beneficial palliatives for juvenile whooping cough.

Lippia Citriodora (Aloysia citriodora)
Also known as Lemon-Scented Verbena
Where grown Throughout the Northern Hemisphere (widely cultivated)
Appearance A procumbent garden plant bearing trusses of brilliant flowers. The dried beans are used.
Therapeutic or culinary uses Its principal use is in cosmetic manufacture, and its essential oil is used as a perfume. It is also a sedative and can be used to expel worms.

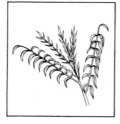

Liquorice (Glycyrrhiza glabra)
Found wild Europe and the Middle East
Appearance A strong-growing perennial plant. The roots are used.
Therapeutic or culinary uses Liquorice is of the greatest value in cough medicines. It is a demulcent and pectoral. It is, as well, a laxative with a gentle action.

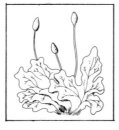

Liverwort (English) (Peltigera canina)
Found wild Throughout Europe
Appearance A small herb. The whole plant is used.
Therapeutic or culinary uses A reliable laxative but if taken in strong doses is a purgative.

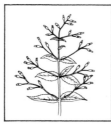

Lobelia (Lobelia inflata)
Found wild United States
Appearance A small herb of trailing habit. The leaves are used.
Therapeutic or culinary uses Lobelia is one of the most valuable and beneficial herbs yet discovered. It is a stimulant and also a diaphoretic and expectorant. It is of great value for the treatment of asthma and whooping cough in children.

Logwood (Haematoxylon campechianum)
Found wild South America
Appearance A large and massive tree. The wood is used.
Therapeutic or culinary uses Logwood is used to relieve diarrhoea and dysentery, and also for women's disorders.

Loosestrife (Lysimachia vulgaris)
Also known as Marsh Loosestrife
Found wild Great Britain, by rivers, streams and marshy places.
Appearance A big busy plant with yellow flowers. The leaves are used.
Therapeutic or culinary uses An astringent, it is principally used to stem an excessive menstrual flow. It can also be used as a gargle to clear the chest.

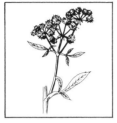

Lovage (Levisticum officinale)
Where found A popular garden plant in Britain.
Appearance A small herb. The root is used.
Therapeutic or culinary uses A carminative. Excellent for relieving flatulence, and soothing to the stomach. It is also a diuretic. When infused it is a valuable complexion wash.

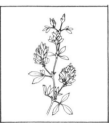

Lucerne (Medicago sativa)
Also known as Alfalfa
Found wild Throughout Europe
Appearance Similar to a large clover. The leaves and stem are used.
Therapeutic or culinary uses It can be taken as an aid to weight increase, particularly by women to increase the size of the breasts. Its principal use, however, is to fatten cattle.

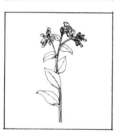

Lungwort (Sticta pulmonaria)
Also known as Lung Moss
Found wild Throughout Europe
Appearance Grey lichen. The lichen is used.
Therapeutic or culinary uses Excellent for the treatment of coughs, asthma and congestion of the lungs. It is also an astringent.
Traditional and/or reputed uses Lungwort was much recommended by the Roman Legion doctors.

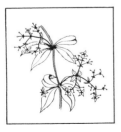

Madder (Rubia tinctorum)
Found wild The Balkans
Appearance A small shrub. All parts are used.
Therapeutic or culinary uses Used for jaundice and spleen complaints.
Traditional and/or reputed uses Much taken by women in ancient times to promote menstruation.

Maidenhair (Adiantum capillus-veneris)
Found wild Europe and Canada
Appearance The most graceful of ferns. The stem and leaves are used.
Therapeutic or culinary uses This makes up into the most effective of hair tonics and is widely used in shampoos. It is an expectorant and pectoral and is very widely used in cough medicines.
Traditional and/or reputed uses Believed in ancient Egypt to be the most certain of all medications to assist the growth of hair.

Malabar-nut (Adhatoda vasica)
Found wild India
Appearance A medium-sized tree. The leaves are used.
Therapeutic or culinary uses It is believed in the East to be the best possible treatment for all chest diseases. It is an expectorant and antispasmodic. Also used in herbal tobacco to relieve asthma.

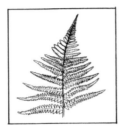

Male Fern (Dryopteris filix-mass)
Also known as Shield Fern
Found wild Europe and the Middle East
Appearance An erect fern of spreading habit. The roots are used.
Therapeutic or culinary uses The male fern is regarded as the remedy most certain to expel tapeworms. It is safe and usually recommended for children.

Manaca (Brunfelsia hopeana)
Found wild South America and West Indies
Appearance A spindly shrub. The roots are used.
Therapeutic or culinary uses An alterative, and of the greatest value for the treatment of arthritis. It eases pain and restores mobility quickly.

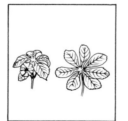

Mandrake (America) (Podophyllum peltatum)
Found wild North America
Appearance A small herb. The rhizomes are used.
Therapeutic or culinary uses This plant is in no way related to the English Mandrake. It chief value is as a long-term general health aid. It cleanses the system and promotes appetite while aiding the digestion.
Traditional and/or reputed uses Was taken daily by Red Indian braves to ensure courage.

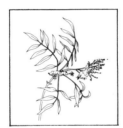

Manna (Fraxinus ornus)
Found wild. Mediterranean countries
Appearance The congealed sap of the manna tree.
Therapeutic or culinary uses A most nutritive invalid food
with a sweet pleasant flavour. It is also used as a gentle
laxative for pregnant women.

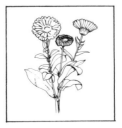

Marigold (Calendula officinalis)
Where found A very popular garden border plant
throughout the Northern Hemisphere
Appearance A small neat plant with show yellow flowers.
The leaves are used.
Therapeutic or culinary uses A stimulant and a diaphoretic,
it was formerly taken to reduce varicose veins. It is little
used now.
Traditional and/or reputed uses The flowers are the altar
offerings of the Hindus.

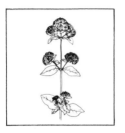

Marjoram, Sweet (Origanum majorana)
Found wild Throughout Europe (also cultivated)
Appearance Commonly grown as a garden plant. The stalks
and leaves are used.
Therapeutic or culinary uses Widely grown as a culinary
seasoning.
Traditional and/or reputed uses Once regarded as a
powerful stimulant

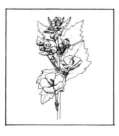

Marshmallow (Althaea officinalis)
Found wild Throughout Europe
Appearance A strong-growing herb with a pronounced
affinity for watery places. The roots and leaves are used.
Therapeutic or culinary uses Its marked emollient and
demulcent properties make it one of the first choices for
incorporation in cough medicines. It is excellent for the
treatment of cystitis and for soothing the alimentary canal.
Authors' comments It is one of the most beneficial of herbs.

Mayweed (Anthemis cotula)
Also known as Dog Fennel
Found wild Throughout Europe
Appearance A low growing herb, a common weed. The
leaves are used.
Therapeutic or culinary uses An antispasmodic with marked
tonic qualities. It is also excellent for migraine.

Meadow Lily (Lilium candidum)
Also known as Madonna Lily
Found wild Europe
Appearance The delightful garden lily. The leaves are used.
Therapeutic or culinary uses This herb is now out of favour for medicinal usage, but in the Middle Ages it was popular for women's disorders. It was also used externally for the treatment of ulcerations and sores.

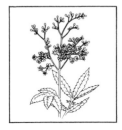

Meadowsweet (Spiraea ulmaria)
Found wild Throughout Great Britain
Appearance A small common herb with tiny yellow flowers. The stem and leaves are used.
Therapeutic or culinary uses An aromatic that was once popular as a flavouring for non-alcoholic drinks. It is a diuretic and excellent for the quick relief of diarrhoea in children.
Traditional and/or reputed uses It was carried during the Great Plague in nosegays to prevent infection

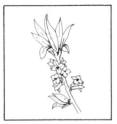

Mezereon (Daphne mesereum)
Also known as Spurge Laurel
Found wild Europe
Appearance A strong, crowded shrub. The bark and root bark and used.
Therapeutic or culinary uses A stimulant, effective for the relief of rheumatism.

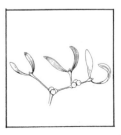

Mistletoe (Viscum album)
Found wild Throughout Europe
Appearance A parasite which grows in the branches of host trees. The leaves are used.
Therapeutic or culinary uses Mistletoe has nervine qualities and is most effective for the treatment of tension, insomnia and depressions. It is also used in larger doses as a narcotic.
Traditional and/or reputed uses It is also used to make 'bird lime'.

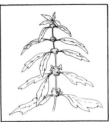

Motherwort (Leonurus cardiaca)
Where found A common garden plant in Britain and throughout Northern Europe.
Appearance A pink-flowered herb of handsome appearance. The leaves are used.
Therapeutic or culinary uses One of the finest of all nervines, especially quick to relieve women's troubles and hysterical upsets. It is also a fine tonic for sufferers from heart diseases, and acts to stimulate the aged and ailing.
Author's comments So efficacious that it is known also as the 'herb of life'.

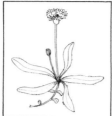

Mouse-Ear (Hieracium pilosella)
Found wild Throughout Europe and Great Britain, growing in sandy places.
Appearance A diminutive trailing herb. The leaves are used.
Therapeutic or culinary uses It is an expectorant and an astringent much used for the relief of lung troubles and whooping cough. It also makes up into an excellent skin salve.
Traditional and/or reputed uses Once much used to temper steel.

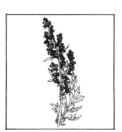

Mugwort (Artemisia vulgaris)
Found wild Throughout Great Britain
Appearance A small herb which profusely seeds itself. The leaves are used.
Therapeutic or culinary uses It is a diuretic and diaphoretic of proven value for bringing on the menses. It is one of the most popular of women's remedies.

Muira-Puama (Liriosma ovata)
Found wild Brazil.
Appearance A tree of considerable size. The roots are used.
Therapeutic or culinary uses One of the strongest and most reliable aphrodisiacs known. It can help prolong virility into extreme old age. Also of great value to women suffering from nervous exhaustion and debility. A stimulant of extraordinary quality.

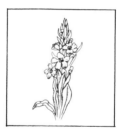

Mullein (Verbascum thapsus)
Found wild Throughout Europe
Appearance A tall perennial plant of cylindrical growth with a tower of yellow flowers. The flowers and leaves are used.
Therapeutic or culinary uses When used as an infusion it is effective for lung and bronchial inflammations. It is an astringent, a demulcent and a pectoral.

Muskseed (Hibiscus abelmoschus)
Found wild India
Appearance A small shrub of bold appearanc. The seeds are used.
Therapeutic or culinary uses An insecticide used since the most ancient times for ridding the body of lice and scabies. Also a strong aromatic used in Thugee religious rites.

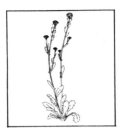

Mustard (Brassica nigra — Black Mustard)
            (Brassica alba — White Mustard)
Found wild Throughout the Northern Hemisphere
Appearance A short-growing annual herb with bright yellow
flowers. The seeds are used.
Therapeutic or culinary uses A powerful irritant and emetic.
Mustard is much used in embrocations for the relief of
rheumatic and arthritic pains, and is added to baths for the
same purpose. It is also famous as a condiment for
negativing the effects of fatty foods.

Myrobalans (Terminalia chebula)
Found wild India
Appearance A moderate to large-sized tree. The fruit is
used.
Therapeutic or culinary uses A reliable cathartic, it also
possesses astringent qualities.
Traditional and/or reputed uses Can be used to tan leather.

Myrrh (Commiphora molmol)
Found wild Arabia and East Africa
Appearance A large shrub of irregular growth. The resinous
hardened gum is used.
Therapeutic or culinary uses Good-quality myrrh is of great
value and is used mostly to perfume temples. It is for
medicinal purposes a valuable stimulant and antiseptic.
Made up into a tincture it is very effective for throat
troubles, ulcers etc.

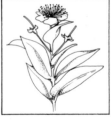

Myrtle (Myrtus communis)
Found wild The warmer areas of Europe
Appearance A strong bushy shrub. The leaves are used.
Therapeutic or culinary uses Once regarded as a cure for
consumption but now often used as a balm for night cramp.

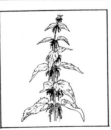

Nettle (Urtica dioica)
Also known as Stinging Nettle
Found wild Grows everywhere in rich soil.
Appearance A hardy perennial with white flowers. The
seeds, flowers and leaves are used.
Therapeutic or culinary uses Nettle is an effective tonic and
promotes are appetite. It is a diuretic and re-invigorates the
liver and kidneys. It rejuvenates the hair and skin when used
as wash.
Authors' comments Persons seeking to purchase a farm
should look for nettles — if there are none, the soil is poor
and hungry.

Night-blooming Cereus (Cereus grandiflorus)
Found wild Jamaica
Appearance A small much branded cactus with large
creamy flowers. All of the plant is used.
Therapeutic or culinary uses A very effective heart
stimulant, best, used for angina pectoris. Excellent for the
quick relief of palpitations. Also a diuretic and can be taken
for prostate diseases with gratifying results.

Nikkar Nuts (Guilandia bondue)
Found wild South America
Appearance A tall slender tree. The seeds are used.
Therapeutic or culinay uses Used regularly by diabetic
sufferers and reported to be effecive. It is also taken to ward
against bouts of malaria.

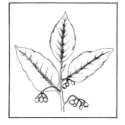

Nutmeg (Myristica fragrans)
Found wild East Indies
Appearance A tree of magnificent growth and habit. The
seeds are used.
Therapeutic or culinary uses A valuable stomachic and
carminative. However, it is chiefly used as a spice. If taken
in abundance it can weaken the system.

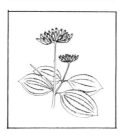

Nux Vomica (Poisonous) (Strychnos nux vomica)
Also known as Poison Nut
Found wild India and the Far East
Appearance A small tree. The seeds are used.
Therapeutic or culinary uses When expertly dispensed the
seeds are an excellent stimulant and general tonic, and are
widely used in medicinal preparations for these purposes.
Authors' comments **Nux Vomica seeds contain Strychnine
and are a dangerous poison.**

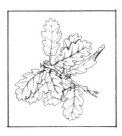

Oak (Quercus robur)
Found wild In most temperate parts of the world
Appearance The massive tree which epitomizes the English
character. The bark is used.
Therapeutic or culinary uses The oak has tonic properties
but is usually prescribed for its astringent qualities. It
relieves diarrhoea and dysentery. Oak bark is commercially
used in the tanning of hides to make leather.

Oats (Avena sativa)
Found wild In most temperate climates
Appearance A common farm crop somewhat similar to
wheat. The seeds are used.
Therapeutic or culinary uses A very effective nerve tonic,
and can allay spasms. Also stimulates the genital organs.

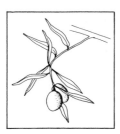

Olive (Olea europaea)
Found wild Mediterranean area
Apperance A gnarled evergreen tree of modest growth and usually giving the appearance of great age. The oil is used.
Therapeutic or culinary uses One of the safest laxatives, sooths and softens the anal passages. It is also much used in the preparation of cosmetics and excellent for the treatment of hair. The fruit when crushed provides the valuable olive oil.

Oliver Bark (Cinnamomum oliveri)
Also known as Australian Cinnamon
Found wild Eastern states of Australia
Appearance A tree of moderate growth, of which the bark is used.
Therapeutic or culinary uses A strong stimulant which promotes endurance. Used by the aborigines to strengthen themselves before beginning their long 'walkabouts'.

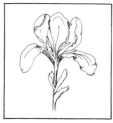

Orris (Iris florentina)
Also known as North Africa
Appearance A sturdy plant like the garden iris. The rhizomes are used.
Therapeutic or culinary uses Effectively relieves bronchial troubles, but is principally used in cosmetic preparations.

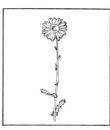

Ox-Eye Daisy (Chrysanthemum leucanthemum)
Also known as Field Daisy
Found wild Europe and Northern Asia
Appearance A very common perennial plant with serrated leaves and white, daisy-like flowers.
Therapeutic or culinary uses The antispasmodic properties of this plant have been recognized throughout history. It relieves whooping cough and asthma and is an effective treatment for female hysteria. It is also a fine tonic.

Papaw (Carica papaya)
Also known as Melon Tree
Found wild Throughout sub-tropical areas
Appearance A tall tree (about 25ft — 8 metres) with boldly serrated leaves. Only the female tree produces fruit. The fruit and leaves are used.
Therapeutic or culinary uses The large fruits, as big as a melon, produce the finest digestive known to science. It is much used in invalid foods and can help clear up duodenal and peptic ulcers. It is also used to tenderize steak.

Paraguay Tea (Ilex paraguensis)
Also known as Mate Tea
Found wild South America
Appearance A dense shrub. The leaves are used.
Therapeutic or culinary uses Mostly used as an infusion.
The caffeine content is very high and it has excellent
stimulant properties. It is frequently used as an aphrodisiac
and more generally as a draught to relieve rheumatism and
arthritis, for which it is claimed to be most effective.
Commonly used to make a most pleasant tea.

Parsley (Carum petroselinum)
Found wild Europe
Appearance Bienniel umbelliferous plant with white flowers
and aromatic leaves. The roots and leaves are used.
Therapeutic or culinary uses Parsley is one of the most
beneficial of all diuretic herbs. It is excellent for the
treatment of all kinds of kidney disorders and is used to
eliminate stones and gravel. Also a strong emmenogogue
and valuable for the treatment of amenorrhoea. One of the
favourite culinary flavourings.

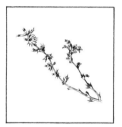

Parsley Piert (Alchemilla arvensis)
Also known Breakstone
Found wild Throughout Europe
Appearance A low-growing herb with tiny green flowers, in
no way related to the common parsley, used for culinary
purposes. The leaves are used.
Therapeutic or culinary uses The most effective medicinal
treatment known for the relief of bladder and kidney
troubles. Is the surest way to dissolve kidney stones

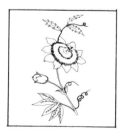

Passion Flower (Passiflora incarnata)
Found wild Throughout the world in warm climates.
Appearance A strong climbing plant with fruits about 3in
(8cm) long. The stems and leaves are used.
Therapeutic or culinary uses A narcotic and sedative with
quick and positive action. Much used to relieve headaches
and migraine and is of great value to women for its
rest-inducing properties. The fruit is used for conserves and
flavouring.

Patchouli (Pogostemon patchouli)
Found wild Malaysia
Appearance A tree with large crenated leaves. The leaves
are used.
Therapeutic or culinary uses Where they can be procured
fresh, the leaves are bruised and spread on floors to arouse
erotic feelings. Also used as a perfume base for cosmetics,
and is imported for this purpose by many countries.

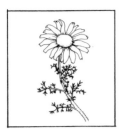

Pellitory (Anacyclus pyrethrum)
Found wild Spain and the South of France
Appearance A small prostrate plant. The root is used.
Therapeutic or culinary uses Used when prepared as a tincture to relieve neuralgia and toothache.
Traditional and/or reputed used The great navigator Vasco da Gama, who had an impacted wisdom tooth, carried it with him on his epic voyage.

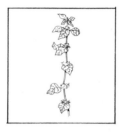

Pellitory-of-the-wall (Parietaria officinalis)
Found wild Throughout Europe
Appearance A herb of medium height with small greenish flowers. The leaves alone are used.
Therapeutic or culinary uses A diuretic with powerful results when used to treat urinary disorders and gravel. As a mild laxative, it is also of use to pregnant women.

Pennyroyal (Mentha pulegium)
Found wild Europe
Appearnce A small herb with a dainty and elegant appearance. The leaves and the oil are used.
Therapeutic or culinary use Chiefly used for its emmenagogue qualities, it is known to be the best and most reliable treatment for obstructed menstruation. It is also a gentle stimulant and diaphoretic.

Peony (Paeonia officinalis)
Found wild Southern Asia
Appearance The beautiful perennial that bears vivid double flowers in profusion.
Therapeutic or culinary uses A proven antispasmodic, once regarded as the best treatment for epilepsy and spasms. Also a tonic recommended for those past middle age.

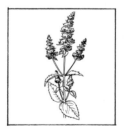

Peppermint (Mintha piperita)
Also known as Curled Mint
Found wild Europe and North America
Appearance A stately herb with purple-hued stems. The leaves and oil are used.
Therapeutic or culinary uses Peppermint is one of the most highly regarded stomachic and carminatives. It relieves all forms of sickness, flatulence and indigestion.
It is also one of the finest flavouring agents known.

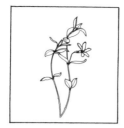

Periwinkle (Vinca major)
Found wild The warmer parts of Europe
Appearance A small decorative herb with delightful blue flowers. The stems and leaves are used.
Therapeutic or culinary uses Chiefly used as a tonic and astringent by women, it is most effective for the treatment of menorrhagia.

Periwinkle (South African) (Vinca rosa)
Found wild South Africa
Appearance A large trailing herb with profuse pink flowers. The stem and leaves are used.
Therapeutic or culinary uses This plant has recently been shown to be an effective treatment for diabetes. Its performance is said to be authoritatively authenticated in South Africa, where it is still the subject of much experimentation.

Peruvian Balsam (Myroxylon pereirae)
Found wild South America
Apperarance A very large tree. The wood is used.
Therapeutic or culinary uses Used as a lotion in cases of eczema, ringworm and skin troubles. It is also a stimulant, and taken as an infusion is excellent for all forms of catarrh and leucorrhoea.

Pichi (Fabiana imbricata)
Found wild South America
Appearance A herb of moderate growth with tiny leaves. The leaves are used.
Therapeutic or culinary uses Pichi is a very effective hepatic and can also be recommended for the treatment of all liver disorders. It is also a stimulant and diuretic and is a reliable treatment for catarrhal and kidney troubles.

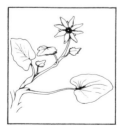

Pilewort (Ranunculus ficaria)
Also known as Lesser Celandine
Found wild Europe; commonly found in Great Britain
Appearance A procumbent yellow-flowered herb. The leaves are used.
Therapeutic or culinary uses Generally regarded as an excellent treatment for piles, for which purpose it is used as both an infusion and an ointment.

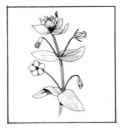

Pimpernel, Scarlet (Poisonous) (Anagallis arvensis)
Found wild Nothern Europe
Appearance A small procumbent plant with vivid red flowers. The leaves are used.
Therapeutic or culinary uses A diuretic and expectorant of value.
Authors' comments **Can be poisonous and should be used with respect.**

Pine Bark (Tsuga canadensis)
Also known as Hemlock Bark
Found wild Canada
Appearance A tall coniferous tree. The bark is used.
Therapeutic or culinary uses A very strong astringent, used by women for the treatment of leucorrhoea.
Traditional and/or reputed uses Excellent for tanning high-grade leather.

Pipsissiwa (Chimaphila umbellata)
Also known as Ground Holly
Found wild Northern Hemisphere
Appearance A small tough shrub. The leaves are used.
Therapeutic or culinary uses A tonic and valuable alterative. Favoured for the treatment of rheumatoid ailments and said to restore mobility quickly. Also effective for those who feel 'run down' and debilitated.

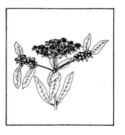

Pleurisy Root (Asclepias tuberosa)
Found wild United States
Appearance A dense shrub of low growth. The roots are used.
Therapeutic or culinary uses Relieves pleurisy by virtue of its remarkable diaphoretic and antispasmodic properties. Also excellent for clearing up catarrh.
Traditional and/or reputed uses An old Red Indian remedy which was much used in patent medicines.

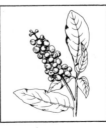

Poke Root (Phytolacca decandra)
Found wild North America
Appearance A shrub with a multitude of grape-sized black berries. The roots and berries are used.
Therapeutic or culinary uses Most frequently used in liquid extract form for the relief of arthritis and rheumatism. It is also an emetic and cathartic.

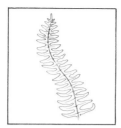

Polypody Root (Polypodium vulgare)
Also known as Brake Root
Found wild Throughout Europe
Appearance A creeping plant attached to tree trunks and walls. The rhizomes and leaves are used.
Therapeutic or culinary uses An expectorant and pectoral and one of the best for the treatment of persistent chest and lung disorders. It is also a good tonic.

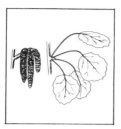

Poplar (Populus tremuloides)
Found wild Throughout Europe
Appearance A very common tree of much elegance. The bark is used.
Therapeutic or culinary uses Usually prescribed for its diuretic qualities. Also a reliable tonic stimulant and formerly much used for this purpose.
Traditional and/or reputed uses Said to be very good for the treatment of debility.

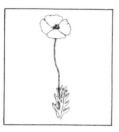

Poppy (Poisonous) (Papaver somniferum)
Found wild Throughout Asia and Europe
Appearance An annual plant with grey leaves and huge, showy single red flowers. Height up to 5ft (2 metres) The seed capsules are used.
Therapeutic or culinary uses The poppy is famous for its ability to ease pain. It is, however, **A Strong Narcotic and should be used only on prescription.**
Authors' comments **This plant is poisonous**

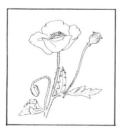

Poppy, Red (Papaver rhoseas)
Also known as Corn Poppy
Found wild Throughout
Appearance This is the common poppy. It grows about 18in (45cm) high and bears bright red single flowers. The flowers are used.
Therapeutic or culinary uses This herb is an efficient anodyne, but it is better known as an expectorant, usually made up with cough mixtures and syrups.

Prickly Ash (Zanthoxylum Americanum)
Found wild North America
Appearance A small tree with long spines. The berries and bark are used.
Therapeutic or culinary uses A stimulant much used for the treatment of rheumatism. Also a diaphoretic and alterative.
Authors' comments It is justly held in the highest regard for its curative properties.

Psylium (Plantago ovata)
Also known as Fleawort
Found wild India
Appearance A small herb. The seeds are used.
Therapeutic or culinary uses When the seeds are soaked they swell into a demulcent mass which, when taken, soothes and cleans the bowels.

Puffball (Lycoperdon bovista)
Found wild Throughout Europe in pastures, healthland and some woods
Appearance A ball-shaped fungus, 4-15in (10-35cm) across, with creamy-white skin.
Therapeutic or culinary uses If burned its smoke has a slight narcotic effect and can be used to stupefy bees.
Traditional and/or reputed uses In Roman times was regarded as effective for staunching blood flow.

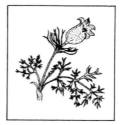

Pulsatilla (Anemone pulsatilla)
Also known as Wind Flower
Found wild Europe
Appearance A large weed with single, anemone-like flowers.
Therapeutic or culinary uses A very useful herb for women with menstruation problems. It is also widely taken to relieve nervous spasms.

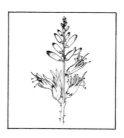

Quassia (Picraena excelsa)
Found wild West Indies
Appearance A tree of great stature. The wood only is used.
Therapeutic or culinary uses Quassia is a good tonic and effective for the treatment of stomach disorders. Also helps sufferers from night cramp.
Traditional and/or reputed uses The West Indies use it for intestinal worms.

Queen's Delight (Stilingia sylvatica)
Also known as Queen's Root
Found wild United States
Appearance A small shrub. The root is used.
Therapeutic or culinary uses The principal constituent in blood-purifying remedies. Can be relied upon to induce a feeling of healthy wellbeing. Also a laxative without any purging effects.

Quince (Cydonia oblongata)
Where found Cultivated throughout Europe
Appearance An ornamental tree of moderate growth. The seeds are used.
Traditional and/or reputed uses Little used in medicine now. In Elizabethan times, quince was recommended for the treatment of dysentery. It was also much used in balm and lotions, for its soothing and whitening qualities.

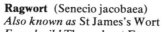

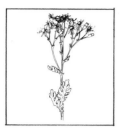

Ragwort (Senecio jacobaea)
Also known as St James's Wort
Found wild Throughout Europe
Appearance An erect slender herb with yellow flowers. The herb is used.
Therapeutic or culinary uses Ragwort is excellent when taken as an infusion for gouty conditions and rheumatic pains. It usually gives great relief quickly. Also very good for lung and bronchial infections. It makes up into a fine ointment for applying to the chest.

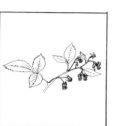

Raspberry (Rubus idaeus)
Where found Under cultivation in most parts of the world
Appearance Produces cane-like growths that are 6-8ft (2-3 metres) in height. Fruits are red and are profuse. The fruit and leaves are used.
Therapeutic or culinary uses A powerful astringent. Can be used with every expectation of success as a mouthwash, and to clean wounds and ulcers.

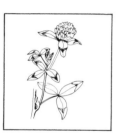

Red Clover (Trifolium pratense)
Also known as Trefoil
Found wild Throughout Europe
Appearance A common clover. All the plant is used.
Therapeutic or culinary uses Used as sedative and to clear up nervous coughs, 'tickling' coughs and whooping cough. It is one of the best herbs to use for children.

Red Sage (Salvia officinalis)
Also known as Sage
Found wild Europe and North America
Appearance A small herb. The leaves are used.
Therapeutic or culinary uses An astringent and most frequently used for sore throats, quinsy and laryngitis. Also a culinary herb.

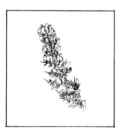

Rest Harrow (Ononis spinosa)
Found wild Throughout Britain
Appearance A very common herb about 2ft (60cm) in height. It is prickly with small purple flowers. The root is used.
Traditional and/or reputed uses A very old diuretic remedy. Also regarded as very helpful for the alleviation of rheumatism.

Rhubarb (Turkey) (Rheum palmatum)
Found wild In China (it does **not** grow in Turkey!)
Appearance A very large, grand variety of rhubarb. The rhizomes are used.
Therapeutic or culinary uses A plant of remarkable properties. It is a fine tonic and an astringent and the best known of purgatives. Very widely used and prescribed.

Rose Red (Rosa gallica)
Also known as French Rose
Found wild The warmer parts of Europe
Appearance A medium sized bush with deep green foliage. The flower petals are used.
Therapeutic or culinary uses As astringent referred to in medieval times as the tonic for lovers. Its principal use now is to provide a base for perfumery. Its hips are one of the most prolific sources of ascorbic acid.
Authors' comments This plant produces the Otto of Roses.

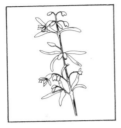

Rosemary (Rosmarinus officinalis)
Found wild Southern Europe and Near East
Appearance A hardy everygreen shrub with fragrant needle-like leaves. The leaves alone are used.
Therapeutic or culinary uses A most satisfying nervine, especially good for persistent headaches and migraine. It is known for promoting hair growth.

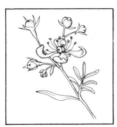

Rue (Dangerous) (Ruta graveolens)
Also known as Garden Rue
Found wild Throughout Europe
Appearance Small hardy evergreen shrub with serrated blush-green leaves. The leaves are used.
Therapeutic or culinary uses Usually prescribed to **suppress** menstruation but can, if taken for several days, prove to be an emmenagogue. It also acts as an antispasmodic.
Traditional and/or reputed uses. Also effective to relieve insect stings.
Authors' comments. **Rue should be taken only in prescribed doses or it can prove harmful.**

Saffron (Crocus sativus)
Found wild East Europe (also cutlivated in England and France)
Appearance A large crocus with a bold flowers. The pistils of the flowers are used.
Therapeutic or culinary uses This is a very costly herb, and is the best and most efficacious emmenagogue known. It is best used for relieving menstrual troubles. it is also much used commercially as a cake flavouring and cloth dye.

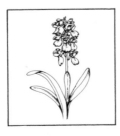

Salep (Orchis mascula)
Found wild Europe and Great Britain
Appearance A strong erect herb. The roots are used.
Therapeutic or culinary uses Salep makes up into excellent invalid food and is regarded as one of the best dietary aids for the senile.
Traditional and/or reputed uses Was once much for kidney disorders.

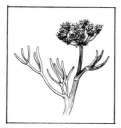

Samphire (Crithmum maritimum)
Also known as Rock Samphire
Found wild England, particularly in saline conditions
Appearance A small herb that prefers the shelter of rocks.
The leaves are used.
Therapeutic or culinary uses Taken by people who want to
lose weight, and considered very effective. Also a diuretic
which has a positive beneficial kidney action.

Sandalwood (Santalum album)
Found wild Malaysia
Appearance An elegant tree of medium size. The wood
raspings are used.
Therapeutic or culinary uses The oil provides one of the
most entrancing perfumes, and is widely used in perfumery
and cosmetics. Medicinally it is a diuretic and of value for
the treatment of bladder inflammation.

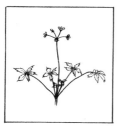

Sanicle (Sanicula europaea)
Also known as Butterwort
Found wild Great Britain
Appearance A small herb with bold green leaves.
Therapeutic or culinary uses As an astringent it is valuable
for relieving leucorrhea.
Traditional and/or reputed uses An old treatment for
dropsy. Also once widely used as a lotion for chilblains and
roughened skin.

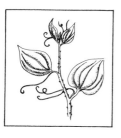

Sarsparilla (Smilax ornata)
Also known as Jamaican Sarsparilla
Found wild South America
Therapeutic or culinary uses An alterative possessing
specific qualities as a blood purifier, and regarded as one of
the best. It is also a very popular health beverage.
Traditional and/or reputed uses Claimed to have
regenerative effects upon the genital organs. Believed by the
Spanish conquerors to be a certain cure for syphillis.

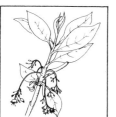

Sassafras (Sassafras variifolium)
Found wild Pacific coast of North America
Appearance A shrub of average size found in mountainous
regions. The bark and roots are used.
Therapeutic or culinary uses A strong stimulant and used by
the American Indians as an aphrodisiac. It is also effective
for arthritis and rheumatism.

Sassy Bark (Poisonous) (Erythrophloeum guineense)
Found wild West Africa
Appearance A small tree of stunted appearance. The bark alone is used.
Therapeutic or culinary uses Has laxative effects but is principally used as a narcotic.
Traditional and/or reputed uses It is much used by witchdoctors who use the smoke from it to stupefy.
Authors' comments **This is poisonous and should only be used when prescribed by an expert.**

Savory Summer (Satureia hortensis)
Where found Commonly cultivated throughout the world as a flavouring herb.
Appearance A small shrubby plant. The leaves are used.
Therapeutic or culinary uses Good for the quick relief of flatulence and indigestion. Also used as a poultice to reduce inflammations.

Saw Palmetto (Serenoa serrulata)
Also known as Sabal
Found wild Pacific coast of North America
Appearance A palm tree of medium growth. The berries are used.
Therapeutic or culinary uses Known to be one of the most effective aphrodisiacs, it is said to preserve virility into old age. It is safe and without irritant effects. It is also a sedative and diuretic.

Scammony Root (Ipomoea orizabnesis)
Found wild Mexico
Appearance A climbing plant with profuse panicles of purple flowers. The roots are used.
Therapeutic or culinary uses Scammony root is one of the most effective purgatives known.

Scopolia (Poisonous) (Scopola carniolica)
Found wild A herb of below-average size. The rhizomes are used.
Therapeutic or culinary uses Used for eye treatments, it is a mydriatic. Also has narcotic properties.
Authors' comments **It is very poisonous and should only be used on prescription.**

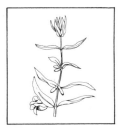

Scullcap (Scutellaria laterifolia)
Found wild United States
Appearance A herb of insignificant appearance with pale blue flowers. The herb is used.
Therapeutic or culinary uses Famous for its qualities as a nervine and tonic, it certainly relieves nervous tension and St Vitus dance. Can be safely taken by persons of any age under any conditions.

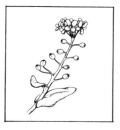

Scurvy-grass (Cochlearia officinalis)
Found wild Southern England
Appearance A small procumbent herb which spreads rapidly. The leaves are used.
Therapeutic or culinary uses Still the most effective method of allaying complexion blemishes.
Traditional and/or reputed uses Scurvy grass was carried on all ships on long passages up to a century ago to prevent scurvy.
Authors' comments Makes up into an excellent gargle as well.

Self-heal (Prunella vulgaris)
Found wild Throughout Great Britain
Appearance A very small prostrate herb with small blue flowers. The leaves are used.
Therapeutic or culinary uses This herb is an astringent and is excellent for throat and bronchial troubles.
Traditional and/or reputed uses Was once used by opera singers and exported to all parts of the world for that purpose.

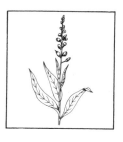

Senega (Polygala senega)
Also known as Senega
Found wild United States
Appearance A low-growing plant with tall flower stems. The roots are used.
Therapeutic or culinary uses A very effective diaphoretic and expectorant. Of great value for the treatment of bronchitis and pneumonia. Asthma sufferers also report very quick relief from its use.

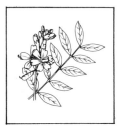

Senna (Cassia angustifolia)
Found wild Arabia
Appearance A tree of sparse growth with distinctive grey-green leaves. The pods are used.
Therapeutic or culinary uses A laxative of high repute. Safe and without purging effects, it is pleasant to take and sure to act.
Authors' comments It is very widely used in ethical medicine preparations.

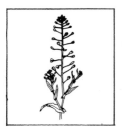

Shepherd's Purse (Capsella bursa-pastoris)
Found wild Everywhere
Appearance A small and quite insignificant weeds with little white flowers. The leaves are used.
Therapeutic or culinary uses It is a diuretic usually taken for kidney and urinary troubles. An antiscorbutic, it prevents scurvy.
Traditional and/or reputed uses Said to be a reliable stimulant, but is little used as such now.

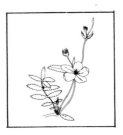

Silverweed (Potentilla anserina)
Also known as Tansy
Found wild Throughout Europe
Appearance A small herb. The leaves are used.
Therapeutic or culinary uses Has been used for centuries as an infusion to eliminate blemishes and faulty skin pigmentation.

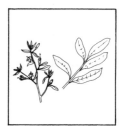

Simaruba (Simaruba amara)
Found wild West Indies
Appearance A tree of less-than-average growth. The bark is used.
Therapeutic or culinary uses Simaruba is one of the finest tonics for persons suffering from debility and loss of appetite.

Skunk Cabbage (Symplocarpus foetidus)
Found wild United States
Appearance A small herb of bulky appearance and foul odour. The leaves are used.
Therapeutic or culinary uses An excellent diaphoretic and expectorant, much used in formulae to reduce temperature and allay fevers. Also regarded as an excellent treatment for influenza.

Slippery Elm (Ulmus fulva)
Found wild North America.
Appearance A great tree of spreading growth. The bark from young saplings is used.
Therapeutic or culinary uses As a nutritive it is the best invalid food known to science. It is also a most valuable emollient and demulcent of the greatest possible healing value for burns and all manner of skin troubles.
Authors' comments Slipper Elm has literally a hundred uses, all of them unexcelled. Demand now exceeds supply.

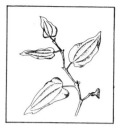

Snake Root (Aristolochia reticulata)
Found wild United States
Appearance A climbing plant with bold white flowers. The rhizomes are used.
Therapeutic or culinary uses A herb with many beneficial uses. It is a stimulant, diaphoretic, antispasmodic, nervine and one of the quickest known anodynes.

Soap Tree (Quillaja saponaria)
Also known as Quillaia Bark
Found wild South America
Appearance A small tree. The bark is used.
Therapeutic or culinary uses Most reliable for soothing and relieving chronic bronchitis and one of the best aids to hair growth, when applied as an infusion to the scalp. Also one of the strongest known sternutatories — it produces sneezing.

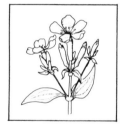

Soapwort (Saponaria officinalis)
Also known as Fuller's Herb (an old name for it)
Found wild Throughout Europe
Appearance A little herb with pink flowers. The roots are used.
Therapeutic or culinary use Used as an infusion it is a very soothing and effective cure for skin diseases. Much used in the brewing industry.

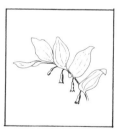

Solomon's Seal (Polygonatum multiflorum)
Where found Throughout Great Britain as a garden plant.
Appearance A tall plant with strap-like leaves and flowers similar to Lily-of-the-Valley. The rhizomes are used.
Therapeutic or culinary uses A demulcent and astringent of considerable value for the alleviation of women's disorders. It also has tonic properties and makes up into a fine complexion lotion.
Therapeutic or culinary uses A demulcent and astringent of considerable value for the alleviation of women's disorders. It also has tonic properties and makes up into a fine complexion lotion.

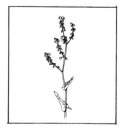

Sorrel (Rumex acetosa)
Found wild In marshy places in Europe
Appearance A small plant with arrow-shaped leaves. The leaves are used.
Therapeutic or culinary uses Excellent for reducing fevers and as a tonic for women, especially during and after menstruation.

Southernwood (Artemisia abrotanum)
Found wild Throughout Europe
Appearance A small herb. The leaves are used.
Therapeutic or culinary uses Southernwood infusions have been taken by women since Roman times to encourage menstruation. It is also a stimulant, although rather weak in its effect.

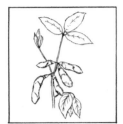

Soya Beans (Glycine max)
Also known as Soybeans
Found wild China
Appearance A tall and strong growing bean. The oil and soy flour are used.
Therapeutic or culinary uses This is one of the most valuable of edible plants but recent discoveries reveal that it has hitherto unsuspected hydrogue qualities, i.e. it can dehydrate the body by voiding water from the tissues.

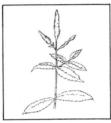

Spearmint (Mentha viridis)
Found wild Throughout the Northern Hemisphere
Appearance A strongly-growing perennial herb. The leaves and oil are used.
Therapeutic or culinary uses A very pleasant stimulant and one of the very best carminatives. Its action is certain and gentle, and is particularly suitable for the very young and the very old.

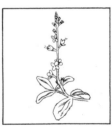

Speedwell (Veronica officinalis)
Also known as European Tea
Found wild Throughout Europe
Appearance A slender tall herb with small blue flowers. The leaves are used.
Therapeutic or culinary uses Although diuretic, it is chiefly used as an expectorant and made up into chest elixirs. As an infusion it is effective when applied to sores and ulcers.
Authors' comments When infused it is also a most delightful tea.

Spikenard (American) (Aralia racemosa)
Found wild North America
Appearance A climbing shrub. The rhizomes are used.
Therapeutic or culinary uses An alterative, and excellent for the treatment of rheumatic disorders. It also has diaphoretic qualities.

Squaw-Vine (Mitchella repens)
Found wild North America
Appearance A small herb of spreading habit. The leaves are used.
Therapeutic or culinary uses Justly regarded as one of the best treatments for the relief of amenorrhoea and menorrhagia, and frequently used for dropsical conditions. It is a diuretic and astingent.

Squill (Urginea maritima)
Found wild Southern Europe and North Africa
Appearance One of the lily family. The bulb is used.
Therapeutic or culinary uses One of the most beneficial
herbs. It is an expectorant and much used in preparations to
relieve catarrh, asthma and bronchial troubles. Also an
excellent cathartic and diuretic.
Authors' comments Squill is used in literally hundreds of
ethical and proprietary medicines.

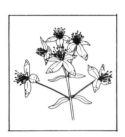

St John's Wort (Hypericum perforatum)
Found wild Great Britain
Appearance A sturdy, yellow-flowered herb. The leaves are
used.
Therapeutic or culinary uses As a diuretic it promotes the
flow of urine. Its expectorant properties make it a most
valuable additive for cough and bronchial medicines.

Stone Root (Collinsonia canadensis)
Found wild Canada
Appearance A small herb. The rhizomes are used.
Therapeutic or culinary uses Although mostly used in
veterinary medicines, it is taken to eliminate bladder stones
and gravel, for which purpose it is regarded as highly
effective.

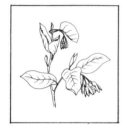

Storax (Liquidambar orientalis)
Also known as Sweet Gum
Found wild Turkey
Appearance A small, sturdy tree. The balsam is used.
Therapeutic or culinary uses Known to be one of the best
expectorants, it is also a powerful stimulant of peculiar
value for its aphrodisiac qualities. Made up into ointments
it can be used for the treatment of scabies and fungus
infections.

Stramonium (Dangerous) (Datura stramonium)
Also known as Thorn Apple
Found wild Europe
Appearance A strong shrub with very beautiful white
trumpet flowers. The leaves and seeds are used.
Therapeutic or culinary uses Stramonium is an anodyne and
narcotic and of great value in the treatment of asthma,
heavy chest colds and lung congestion. It is also used as an
ointment to relieve external inflammation.
Authors' comments **This herb should be used with great
caution!**

Strophanthus (Poisonous) (Strophanthus kombe)
Found wild East Africa
Appearance A climbing plant. The seeds are used.
Therapeutic or culinary uses One of the strongest cardiac
tonics known.
Authors' comments **Should be taken only when expertly
prescribed. It is very poisonous.**

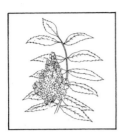

Sumach (Rhus aromatica)
Also known as Sweet Sumach
Found wild North America
Appearance A straggling shrub. The bark from the roots is used.
Therapeutic or culinary uses Sumach is a strong diuretic and used to clear up vaginal discharges. It is also effective when taken by sufferers from incontinence, and helps to clear up this distressing disorder.

Sumbul (Ferula sumbul)
Also known as Musk Root
Found wild East Asia
Appearance A shrub of moderate growth. The root is used.
Therapeutic or culinary uses A very effective nerve stimulant and tonic. Also used to allay female disorders.

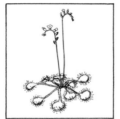

Sundew (Drosera rotundifolia)
Found wild Europe, in marshy places.
Appearance A small plant which traps flies and small insects and digests them.
Therapeutic or culinary uses A pectorant and demulcent of great efficiency in the treatment of troublesome, long-continuing chest troubles.

Swamp Milkweed (Asclepias incarnata)
Found wild United States
Appearance A medium-sized shrub of grotesque appearance. The roots and rhizomes are used.
Therapeutic or culinary uses It is a cathartic and is beneficial in the treatment of arthritis and stomach disorders. Can also be used as an emetic.

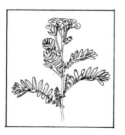

Tansy (Tanacetum vulgare)
Found wild Europe
Appearance A small herb. The leaves are used.
Therapeutic or culinary uses Tansy is one of the oldest known anthelmintics and is now usually used to rid children of worms. It is a reliable emmenagogue and valuable for the treatment of women's disorders.

Thuja (Thuja occidentalis)
Also known as Arbor Vitae
Found wild Canada
Appearance A spreading conifer of small stature. The leaves are used.
Therapeutic or culinary uses An irritant and emmenagogue. Good for the treatment of fevers, coughs and ammennorrhoea. Can also be used as an ointment for the removal of warts.

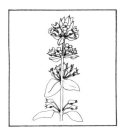

Thyme (Thymus vulgaris)
Also known as Garden Thyme
Found wild Throughout Europe
Appearance A small aromatic perennial herb with violet flowers. The stem and leaves are used.
Therapeutic or culinary uses Thyme is used in medicine as an antispasmodic and antiseptic, mostly for lung troubles.

Tonka Beans (Dangerous) (Dipteryx odorata)
Found wild South America
Appearance A large annual herb of the pea family. The beans are used.
Therapeutic or culinary uses Used as a heart tonic, it has very strong narcotic properties. Much used in the cosmetics industry, as the seeds are delightfully aromatic.
Authors' comments **Should only be taken when prescribed.**

Tragacanth (Astragalus gummifer)
Also known as Gum Tragacanth
Found wild Near East
Appearance A shrub with long thorns. The gum is used.
Therapeutic or culinary uses Used to make up lozenges and emulsions. Frequently used also to allay diarrhoea.

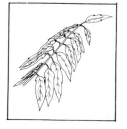

Tree Of Heaven (Ailanthus glandulosa)
Found wild Europe
Appearance A tall and noble tree. The bark is used.
Traditional and/or reputed uses Little used now, it was once highly regarded for the treatment of dysentery and leucorrhoea. It is unpleasant to take.

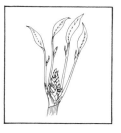

Turmeric (Curcuma longa)
Found wild Asia
Appearance A sturdy herb. The rhizomes are used.
Therapeutic or culinary uses It is cultivated to make curry powder.
Traditional and/or reputed uses Very quickly relieves flatulence and indigestion and was regarded as an excellent liver tonic, but is not much used medicinally nowadays.

Unicorn Root (False) (Chamaelirium luteum)
Found wild United State.
Appearance A tall herb of the lily family. The rhizomes are used.
Therapeutic or culinary uses A tonic, excellent for minor stomach troubles and a diuretic of value for the treatment of kidney troubles. It is effective for spermatorrhoea.
Authors' comments It is popular commercially because of the rarity and very high cost of the true unicorn root (Aletris farinosa).

Unicorn Root (True) (Aletris farinosa)
Also known as Colic Root
Found wild United States
Appearance Another herb of the lily family. The rhizomes are used.
Therapeutic or culinary uses Known to be one of the best tonics for female use — excellent for loss of virility and for debility and troubles arising from the menopause. Also an extremely effective stomachic.

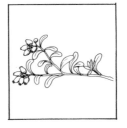

Uva-Ursi (Arctostaphylos uva-ursi)
Found wild Europe and North America
Appearance A small evergreen shrub. The leaves are used.
Therapeutic or culinary uses This excellent herb is one of the best diuretics and of importance for the treatment of urinary troubles. It is much used for relieving menorrhagia and leucorrhoea.

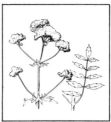

Valerian (Valeriana officialis)
Found wild Great Britain in marshy areas
Appearance A small herb. The rhizomes are used.
Therapeutic or culinary uses Valerian is a nervine of extraordivary virtues. It is very effective for relieving nervous tension or nervous debility, and is excellent when used as a soporific. One of the best anodynes.

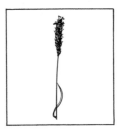

Vernal Grass, Sweet (Anthoxanthum odoratum)
Found wild Europe
Appearance One of the grass family. The flowers are used.
Therapeutic or culinary uses A useful expectorant when made up into gargles and sprays. Also a good scalp cleanser and hair tonic.

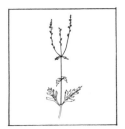

Vervain (Verbena officinalis)
Found wild Great Britain
Appearance Small trailing herb with pink flowers. The leaves are used.
Therapeutic or culinary uses Vervain is a fine nervine and relieves depressions and anxiety neurosis. Also an emetic and a sudorific, i.e. a substance that induces heavy perspiration.

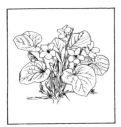

Violet (Viola odorata)
Also known as Sweet Violet
Found wild Europe
Appearance The small wild violet. The flowers and leaves are used
Therapeutic or culinary uses A most effective expectorant, frequently made up into elixirs and syrups. It also has remarkable antiseptic properties.

Wahoo (Euonymus atropurpureus)
Also known as Euonymus
Found wild United States
Appearance A small tree. The bark is used.
Therapeutic or culinary uses Its powerful cholagogue qualities make it one of the most effective aids for the alleviation of liver troubles. It is also a mild laxative and alterative.

Wake Robin (American) (Arum triphyllum)
Found wild United States
Appearance One of the arum lily family; grows in bold clumps. The root is used.
Therapeutic or culinary uses An expectorant used in cough medicines to relieve coughs, colds and lung congestion.

Water Betony (Scrophularia aquatica)
Found wild Throughout Europe
Appearance A herb of medium size that grows beside water. Only the leaves are used.
Therapeutic or culinary uses Used in ointment and poultices for skin complaints. An excellent vulnerary.
Traditional and/or reputed uses Used in more violent times as a specific for healing battle wounds.

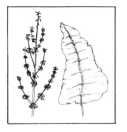

Water Dock (Rumex aquaticus)
Also known as Bloodwort
Found wild Throughout Europe
Appearance One of the common dock family and a water-lover. The roots are used.
Therapeutic or culinary uses Principally used now as a gargle to clean and strengthen the gums and relieve mouth ulcers. It is a detergent and an alterative.

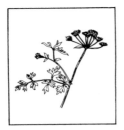

Water Dropwort (Poisonous) (Oenanthe crocata)
Found wild Europe
Appearance A small herb that grows besides running water.
The root is used.
Traditional and/or reputed uses Said to be effective for the
treatment of hysteria.
Authors' comments **It is deadly poisonous and should be
taken only when prescribed by an expert.**

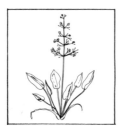

Water Plantain (Alisma plantago)
Found wild Throughout Europe
Appearance A small herb with strap-like leaves which
thrives by running water. The leaves are used.
Therapeutic or culinary uses A diuretic of proven value for
the treatment of gravel and kidney stones. Also excellent for
the treatment of feverish conditions, when taken as an
infusion.

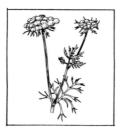

Wild Carrot (Daucus carota)
Found wild Europe
Appearance A small herb with finely serrated typical carrot
leaves. The leaves are used.
Therapeutic or culinary uses A gentle stimulant of peculiar
benefit to the obese. Also a diuretic that quickly relieves
bladder troubles and corrects fluid retention.

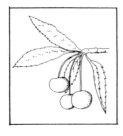

Wild Cherry (Prunus serotina)
Found wild North America
Appearance A small tree. The bark is used.
Therapeutic or culinary uses An excellent tonic for those
recovering from chest troubles. It is it's pectoral qualities
that make it famous: It is one of the more reliable
treatments for lung congestion and whooping cough.

Wild Mint (Mentha sativa)
Also known as Marsh Mint
Found wild Throughout Europe
Appearance Similar to garden mint. The leaves are used.
Therapeutic or culinary uses An astringent, a gentle
stimulant and a strong emetic. Of great aid to women who
suffer from menstrual flooding.

Willow, American Black (Salix discolor)
Found wild United States
Appearance A typical willow tree. The bark is used.
Therapeutic or culinary uses This has quite extraordinary
powers to lessen the sexual libido. It is effective for
controlling night emissions and premature ejaculation.
Makes up into a soothing poultice for varicose ulcers and
has excellent healing properties.

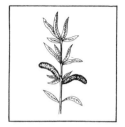

Willow, White (Salix alba)
Also known as Common Willow
Found wild Europe
Appearance The tree that grows by streams and rivers. The
bark and leaves are used
Therapeutic or culinary uses A tonic that relieves rheumatic
and arthritic conditions. Also an antiperiodic, i.e. prevent
the recurrence of certain diseases, particularly malarial
bouts.
Traditional and/or reputed uses Was once much used as a
bath additive. It also thoroughly cleanses the scalp.

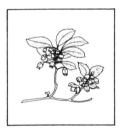

Wintergreen (Gaultheria procumbens)
Found wild North America
Appearance A small procumbent shrub. The leaves are used
Therapeutic or culinary uses Wintergreen is an astringent
and controls diarrhoea, but it is chiefly used for its
stimulant qualities. It is one of the best remedies for
rheumatism known. Also used in embrocations for
sportsmen. Its aromatic odour is very well known.

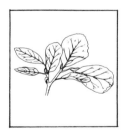

Witch Hazel (Hamamelis virginiana)
Found wild United States
Appearance A slender tree of modest growth. The bark and
leaves are used.
Therapeutic or culinary uses One of the most beneficial of
curative herbs. It is a sedative, a tonic and an astringent. It
is very successful for the treatment of piles and
haemorrhages. It is also much used in ointments for the
treatment of varicose ulcers, and for hair and scalp troubles.

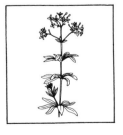

Woodruff (Asperula odorata)
Found wild Throughout Great Britain and Europe
Appearance A small herb that prefers shade. The leaves are
used.
Therapeutic or culinary uses A tonic of particular value for
liver disorders. A diuretic, useful for the treatment of
prostate troubles.

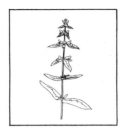

Woundwort (Stachys palustris)
Found wild Great Britain
Appearance A diminutive herb. The leaves are used.
Therapeutic or culinary uses An antispasmodic, used to relieve night cramps and giddiness. Its name relates to its high reputation for healing wounds rapidly.

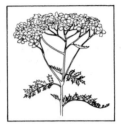

Yarrow (Achillea millefolium)
Also known as Milfoil
Found wild Great Britain
Appearance A tiny herb. The leaves only are used.
Therapeutic or culinary uses A stimulant and diaphoretic. Excellent for the treatment of influenza and heavy chest colds. Much used in blood-purifying compounds.
Traditional and/or reputed uses It is **incorrectly** supposed to be effective for the treatment of rheumatic disorders.

Yellow Parilla (Menispermum canadense)
Found wild North America
Appearance A shrub of prostrate growth. The root is used.
Therapeutic or culinary uses An effective tonic that restores appetite and energy. Increased dosage has a laxative action. Also a reliable treatment for blood disordes and boils.

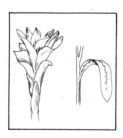

Zedoary (Curcuma zedoaria)
Found wild India
Appearance A herb of modest growth. The rhizomes are used.
Therapeutic or culinary uses A mild stimulant that acts upon the stomach to ease flatulence and aid digestion.
Authors' comments Referred to in ancient books as 'The Banquet Herb'.